Death by Regulation

Also by Mary J. Ruwart, PhD:

Healing Our World (1992, 1993, 2003, 2015)
Lethal Compassion: Why Government Medicine Is the Cure that Kills
(with Jarret Wollstein, 1994)
Short Answers to the Tough Questions (1998, 2012)

Death by Regulation

How We Were Robbed of a Golden Age of Health and How We Can Reclaim It

by Mary J. Ruwart, PhD

SunStar Press and Liberty International
Kalamazoo, MI, and San Francisco, CA

Published jointly by:

SunStar Press   Liberty International
3802 Franklin   237 Kearny Street
Kalamazoo, MI 49001-4149   San Francisco, CA 94108-4502

ISBN: 978-0-9632336-1-5

Library of Congress Cataloging-in-Publication Data

Names: Ruwart, Mary J., author.
Title: Death by regulation : how we were robbed of a golden age of health
  and how we can reclaim it / by Mary J. Ruwart.
Description: Kalamazoo, MI : SunStar Press ; San Francisco, CA : Liberty
  International, [2018] | Includes bibliographical references and index.
Identifiers: LCCN 2018008428 (print) | LCCN 2018010305 (ebook) | ISBN
  9780963233639 | ISBN 9780963233615
Subjects: | MESH: Legislation, Drug | Health Care Reform | United States
Classification: LCC RA771.5 (ebook) | LCC RA771.5 (print) | NLM QV 33 AA1 |
  DDC 362.1/0425--dc23
LC record available at https://lccn.loc.gov/2018008428

Contents

Abbreviations ix

Foreword xi

Preface xiv

1. The Life You Save May Be Your Own 1

2. The Thalidomide Tragedy Created an Even Bigger One. 7

3. The FDA Is Given Carte Blanche 11

4. A Revolving Door Swings between Drug Companies
    and the FDA 16

5. Is "Safe and Effective" a Myth? 23

6. The FDA Becomes the Scapegoat. 28

7. AIDS Patients Take Matters into Their Own Hands 32

8. Courts Rule We Can't Save Our Lives with Unapproved Drugs 35

9. Americans Die Waiting While Brits Enjoy "Made in America" Drugs
    First. 38

10. Millions of Americans Die Waiting for Lifesaving Drugs. 43

11. What Takes So Long? 48

12. The Amendments Put Small Firms Out of Business 56

13. Rules Are for Thee, But Not for Me 61

14. Congress Acknowledges Regulations Account for Half
    of Drug Development Time 73

15. Lifesaving Information for Older Drugs Is Delayed 75

16. Off-Label Use Shows How the Market Can
    Determine Effectiveness 80

17. Development Costs Skyrocket 84

18. Regulatory Costs Determine What You Pay at the Pharmacy 88

19. What Would Drug Prices Have Been Without the Amendments? 92

20. How Have the Amendments Enabled the Greedy? 97

21. Innovation Is Imperative 101

22. The Amendments Slashed Innovation by Pharmaceutical Firms 105

23. Innovation Is Thwarted by the Amendments. 107

24. The Amendments Have Destroyed About 80%
    of Our Innovations 110

25. Britain Does It Better 115

26. Innovators Lose Even When They Succeed 117

27. Loss of Innovation Means Shorter Lives 121

28. Loss of Pharmaceutical Innovation Means Higher
    Health Care Costs. 124

29. The Amendments Stifled Innovation by Physicians:
    Stem Cell Research 127

30. The Amendments Stifled Innovation by Physicians:
    Cancer Treatments 132

31. The Costs of the Amendments Are Not Offset by
    Their Benefits 138

32. The Amendments Shift Our Medical Paradigm from
    Prevention to Treatment 157

33. Expensive Drugs Are Now Replacing Affordable
    Natural Products. 161

34. The Amendments Are Responsible for the
    "American Thalidomide" 163

35. Information about Nutrition Is a Matter of Life and Death 166

36. The Amendments Restrict Information about Prevention.......... 171

37. The FDA Raids Stores and Physicians Promoting Prevention....... 175

38. The FDA Refuses to Obey Courts Orders....................... 179

39. The FDA Turns Foods into Drugs 182

40. Supplements Make Drugs Safer 186

41. Inexpensive Prevention Becomes Expensive Treatment........... 189

42. New Dietary Ingredients Regulations Thwart Prevention 192

43. Thalidomide Takes Us Back to the Future 195

44. How the Amendments Have Institutionalized Corruption 197

45. The Amendments Are a Cure Worse than the "Disease" 200

46. We Are All Hamed by the Amendments....................... 207

47. What Would We Have Had without the Amendments?........... 209

48. Where Did the Amendments Go Wrong?...................... 212

49. How Do We Fix the Problems Caused by the Amendments? 215

50. Certification Is the Alternative to Regulation................... 222

51. Drug Companies Rarely Profit by Selling Unsafe
    or Ineffective Drugs 229

52. Would Drug Development Change without
    FDA Approval? 232

Afterword 240

Acknowledgments 244

Endnotes 247

References 250

Index 285

About the Author... 302

DEDICATION

This book is dedicated to the millions throughout the world who have died prematurely because of the deadly side effects of pharmaceutical regulations—and the millions more who are dying at this very moment.

Abbreviations and Acronyms

AHFS	American Hospital Formulary Service
AIDS	acquired immune deficiency syndrome
ALS	amyotrophic lateral sclerosis, or Lou Gehrig's disease
AMA	American Medical Association
AMD	age-related macular degeneration
ANDA	Abbreviated New Drug Application
ANP	atrial natriuretic peptide
AZT	azidothymidine
BHRT	bioidentical hormone replacement therapy
CDC	Centers for Disease Control and Prevention
CEO	Chief Executive Officer
CMV	cytomegalovirus retinitis
CoQ10	Coenzyme Q10
DCB	device certifying body
ddC	Zalcitabine (2'-3'-dideoxycytidine)
DHA	docosahexaenoic acid
DNA	deoxyribonucleic acid
DSHEA	Dietary Supplement Health and Education Act of 1994
EPA	eicosapentaenoic acid
FDA	Food and Drug Administration

GDP	gross domestic product
GMP	Good Manufacturing Practices
HIV	human immunodeficiency virus
HRT	hormone replacement therapy
INDs	investigational new drugs
IRB	Institutional Review Board
LD50	lethal dose of an ingested substance that kills 50% of a test sample
LEF	Life Extension Foundation
MI	myocardial infarction, or heart attack
MRSA	methicillin-resistant Staphylococcus aureus
MS	multiple sclerosis
NBEs	new biologically based entities
NCEs	new chemical entities
NCI	National Cancer Institute
NDA	New Drug Application
NDI	new dietary ingredients
NIH	National Institutes of Health
NLEA	Nutrition Labeling and Education Act of 1990
NMEs	new molecular entities
OAM	Office of Alternative Medicine
PCBs	polychlorinated biphenyls
PCP	Pneumocystis pneumonia
PDUFA	Prescription Drug User Fee Act
PGE1	Prostaglandin E1
PMA	Pharmaceutical Manufacturers' Association
PRRT	Peptide Receptor Radionuclide Therapy
R&D	research and development
RDA	recommended daily allowance
RSV	respiratory syncytial virus
UK	United Kingdom
UL	Underwriters Laboratories Inc.

Foreword

Most Americans believe that consumer protection regulation actually keeps them from harm. Unfortunately, that is rarely, if ever, the case. The 1962 Amendments to the Food and Drug Act, which were supposed to keep the American public safe from dangerous drugs like thalidomide, have actually done just the opposite. In *Death by Regulation*, Dr. Ruwart shows us that bad laws can have side effects that are just as deadly as pharmaceutical drugs. Indeed, she suggests that we have each probably lost years of our lives because of the Amendments.

When I served my many terms in Congress, I was able to see first hand how the Amendments empowered the pharmaceutical cartel, gave the Food and Drug Administration (FDA) the power to deny Americans access to promising new drugs, and kept Americans from learning about how to prevent disease. As a physician, I found this assault on prevention especially troubling.

To at least partially counter the deadly side effects of the Amendments, I regularly introduced legislation (The Health Freedom Act) to prevent the FDA from censoring truthful claims about the health benefits of foods and dietary supplements. This legislation would have restored the First Amendment to commercial speech, something that the FDA claims isn't protected by our Constitution. While I was advancing this bill, several federal courts ruled that the FDA's censorship of truthful health claims violated the First Amendment! However, as Dr. Ruwart describes, the FDA managed to have this ruling overturned, courtesy of the power bestowed on it by the Amendments.

Anyone who believed the small government rhetoric of the Republicans who controlled Congress during most of my tenure would have expected my health freedom legislation to sail through the House and Senate. However, this pro-liberty, pro-consumer legislation was all but ignored by the congressional leadership.

My legislation to repeal the FDA's prohibition on drinking raw milk was also disregarded. The major opposition to raw milk was big agribusiness. Large dairy producers want to squelch competition from the small farmers who sell unpasteurized milk.

My experience in Congress supports Dr. Ruwart's assertion that most "consumer protection" legislation actually protects big business to the detriment of its smaller competitors. In the process, consumers lose some of their choices, pay higher prices, and are stuck with fewer options than they otherwise would have had.

The cost of fewer options in pharmaceuticals, medical breakthroughs, or prevention is not just in dollars, but in loss of life. Using data from a number of published studies, Dr. Ruwart conservatively estimates that at least half of the Americans who have died since 1962 have lost more than a decade of their lives because of the Amendments. A more realistic estimate is that we all have lost years that we otherwise would have had with our families, friends, and colleagues.

That is why books like *Death by Regulation: How We Were Robbed of a Golden Age of Health and How We Can Reclaim It* are so important. Dr. Ruwart's inside account of how well-intended legislation actually harms consumers while empowering politicians, bureaucrats, and the very interests that the legislation was supposed to regulate shows why ending the FDA's stranglehold on health care freedom will give us longer and healthier lives.

While I was serving in Congress, Dr. Ruwart was working at Upjohn, a drug company known for its ground-breaking research. Step-by-step, she shows how the Amendments, even today, are re-shaping the FDA, the drug industry, and the field of medical practice, while shifting us away from a prevention paradigm to a treatment-based one. You'll want to read this book carefully: your life may depend on it.

—Ron Paul, MD
Former US Representative from Texas;
former candidate for US President
http://www.ronppaullibertyreport.com
http://ronpaulinstitute.org

Preface

In this extremely well-documented book, Dr. Mary Ruwart explains that too many of us in our "free" country are dying because of federal laws—the 1962 Amendments to the Food & Drug Act—that were supposed to protect us from harm. *Death by Regulation* is—sadly—an accurate title.

For example, in the 1970s, Dr. Stanislaw Burzynski started treating human cancers with natural substances (antineoplastons) normally found in the bodies of humans who don't have cancer. Individuals afflicted with brain cancers had higher chances of cure with fewer adverse effects than with any conventional or "standard of care" brain cancer treatments. In Chapter 30, Dr. Ruwart describes the decades-long persecution of Dr. Burzynski under the Amendments for his "crime" of trying to use those natural protein fragments to cure the deadly cancers.

In July 2014, an MD friend of mine applied for "permission" from the Food and Drug Administration (FDA) to use the Burzynski treatment for a child suffering from an inoperable brain cancer. The antineoplaston therapy is being studied under FDA-sanctioned protocols but may never be approved because of the regulatory road blocks driven by the Amendments and described in this book.

The FDA responded: "A review of the data ... does not support a finding that the potential benefits justify the potential risks of the treatment use in this patient.... [Y]ou must provide evidence that would support a finding that the potential benefits from antineoplaston treatment justify the potential risks."

What's this? Dr. Burzynski's therapy—using molecules present in cancer-free human bodies, molecules that have a solid record since 1976 of curing a significant percentage of brain cancers without significant harm—was judged by FDA personnel to be *more dangerous than dying from brain cancer!* Denied access to a treatment that might have cured his brain cancer and having had no help from the "standard of care," the child died. That's just one example of how "death by regulation" can happen.

It's so very, very sad that despite our right to life, liberty, and the pursuit of happiness, we are forced to beg bureaucrats for permission to save our own lives when all "approved" remedies have failed—and even worse, that permission can be denied!

As Dr. Ruwart details in this book, jumping through the regulatory hoops is very expensive. Those costs cause drug prices to skyrocket without adding significantly to treatment safety. Since the 1990s, I have personally spoken with—and in some cases observed—many individuals who have cured their own skin cancers with a very safe, natural remedy that's not FDA "approved" and so must be obtained outside our "free country." Those skin cancers are cured without a physician, without surgery, and within two to four months with this very well-researched natural treatment. No kidding!

Unfortunately, this safe and effective skin cancer cure was banned— thanks to the Amendments—years ago when it was offered for sale in our "free country" by Lane Laboratories, which was also punished with millions of dollars in fines. Anyone who wants to use it must order it from outside the borders of the "land of the free." (For complete information about this natural skin cancer cure—in readable English—see the books *The Eggplant Cancer Cure* and *Inspired by Nature, Proven by Science,* both written by Bill Cham, PhD, or go to www.curaderm.net).

In *Death by Regulation*, Dr. Ruwart shows how the Amendments cre-ated limitations on the American public's access to information about how very important vitamins, minerals, and other natural substances are to our health. Dr. Ruwart describes how suppression of health-saving in-formation has moved us from a medical paradigm that emphasizes treat-ment instead of prevention. The FDA's armed raids on my office, health food stores, and supplement retailers (Chapter 37) had a chilling effect on the business of keeping us well.

In Chapter 19, Dr. Ruwart introduces us to compounding pharma-cies. She uses their pricing of two natural hormones to demonstrate that the Amendment-driven regulatory requirements drive drug prices up about 40-fold. Using the power bestowed on it by the Amendments, the FDA is now attempting to limit or remove natural hormones that women use to treat menopause (often called "bioidentical hormones," or BHRT for bioidentical hormone replacement therapy) from the market. Should that happen, women who want to use bioidentical hormones will no lon-ger be able to get them. They will either have to suffer the negative effects of menopause or take hormones that are unnatural to the human female (often called "hormone replacement therapy," or HRT) and that are mar-keted by the drug industry instead. Some of those unnatural hormones, such as the synthetic progestins, may increase the risk of breast cancer.

Indeed, many pharmacists and doctors are concerned that the FDA is attempting to destroy compounding pharmacies themselves. Two CEOs of such establishments confirmed that the FDA is trying to put those naturally occurring hormones on the "dangerous" list and force com-pounding pharmacies to build "clean rooms" for "safety." Since 1982, no pharmacist has ever, ever reported any injury caused by compounding the natural hormones used for BHRT. However, the clean rooms will cost about a quarter of a million dollars, which will double or triple the cost of BHRT! Several smaller compounding pharmacies have already closed in anticipation of this forced action.

Should the FDA drive compounding pharmacies from the market, your physician will no longer be able to prescribe—and pharmacies will no longer be able to provide—medicines that are made specifically for you. For example, if you are allergic to some ingredients in medications that you need, your pharmacist will no longer be able to customize them for you. You can read more about this particular concern at http://www.anh-usa.org/protect-natural-estriol/. The Alliance for Natural Health (http://www.ahn-usa.org) informs the American public about regulation and legislation that could compromise health, and it gives us a quick and inexpensive way to push back against such threats. Membership is free.

I could go on and on about all the deaths, enormous health care costs, and suffering caused by the Amendments as well as the regulation, legislation, court decisions, and threats to our health that they continue to spawn, but that's covered very, very well by Dr. Ruwart in the following pages. In *Death by Regulation*, Dr. Ruwart has done a terrific job of researching and explaining to us why the title of this book is entirely but very sadly true. Thank you, Dr. Ruwart!

—jonathan v. wright md, nd (honorary)
tahomaclinic.com
www.greenmedicinenewsletter.com
www.greenmedicineonline.com

Chapter 1

The Life You Save
May Be Your Own

I was just a child when the heart-rending pictures of thalidomide babies, missing one or more limbs, appeared in *Life Magazine*. Their
deformities were caused by a new drug, thalidomide, which their
mothers had taken in early pregnancy, usually to lessen their morning
sickness. Those deformities evoked deep compassion in me. Even at my
young age, I knew such children would have a more difficult life than
would youngsters with normal limbs.

The company that made the drug had not tested it in pregnant
animals before marketing it. Because the deformed babies were born
many months after the drug was taken, thousands of babies were ir-
reversibly harmed before the drug's devastating effects were realized.
Most of the children were European, because the Food and Drug Administration (FDA) had not yet approved thalidomide for sale in the
United States.

However, a few American doctors did have thalidomide samples,
which drug companies routinely and legally gave out to provide safety
data for FDA approval. Consequently, 17 US babies were born with missing limbs (Bren 2001).

In response to this tragedy, Congress enacted the 1962 Kefauver-Harris Amendments to the 1938 Food and Drug Act. Like many other

Americans, my family and I felt reassured that these laws would prevent future drug disasters.

The intent of the Amendments was to protect the American public. Unfortunately, new laws, like new drugs, often have deadly side effects. Behind the scenes, the 1962 Amendments reshaped the pharmaceutical, nutritional, and medical industries in ways detrimental to our health and longevity. Because of the way they were written, the Amendments continue to metastasize into those three areas today. Almost all drug-related legislation passed since then has attempted, with limited success, to correct the ever-growing problems created by the Amendments. The deadly side effects of the Amendments have likely cost each one of us many years of life.

Americans are literally dying for fundamental reform of drug regulation.
—Dr. Henry I. Miller, Founding Director of the Office of Biotechnology, FDA

What specifically did the Amendments do? They gave the FDA the power to decide which animal safety studies the drug companies had to do before the drugs could be tested in people. The FDA could determine what human studies were necessary for it to approve a drug as "safe and effective." Before the Amendments, a drug had needed only to be shown "safe for the intended use." Once a drug company asked the FDA to approve a drug, someone at the agency had to "sign off" rather than simply let 6 months elapse without objection.

The FDA could determine manufacturing standards for the new drug and do inspections to ensure that its dictates were met. Furthermore, the FDA was given jurisdiction over all pharmaceutical advertising as well (US Code 1962). In other words, the FDA was given unprecedented control over the entire drug development process in the hopes that drugs not only would be safe but also would be effective, advertised accurately, and manufactured carefully.

What the Amendments actually did was increase the time it takes for a new drug to move from the lab bench to the marketplace: a change from

4 years to 14 years over the next several decades (Chapter 6). Terminally ill patients who couldn't live with that delay turned to the black market to get access to potential cures (Chapter 7). Every year, the costs of satisfying the FDA have soared (Chapter 17), resulting in ever-increasing prices at the pharmacy (Chapter 18). More than half of our potential innovations have never made it to patients because companies realized they couldn't recoup their investments under the new regulations (Chapters 21–24).

Ironically, the Amendments created an "American thalidomide" by sentencing thousands of US infants to life in an institution; some would be aborted when their deformities were detected in early pregnancy. The press and public would be largely unaware that those birth defects—more horrific and numerous than the European thalidomide tragedy—were preventable. Few would be aware that the 1962 Amendments, passed to keep such a tragedy from happening, had actually created it (Chapter 34).

Losses of innovations and delays in the ones we do get have caused the premature death of almost half of the Americans who have died from disease since 1962 (Chapter 27). By discouraging the use of inexpensive supplements in favor of FDA-approved pharmaceuticals, the Amendments shifted the health care paradigm in the United States from inexpensive prevention to costly treatment (Chapters 32–42). The loss in lives and money from this shift is probably higher than the devastating cost of the Amendment-driven reshaping of medical practice and of the pharmaceutical industry because each one of us has been adversely affected.

The unintended consequences of the Amendments went far beyond the United States. Because most of the medical, pharmaceutical, and nutritional research occurred in the United States, the devastating consequences have rippled outward to affect the entire world.

In the 1960s, humanity was poised on the brink of a Golden Age of Health. Infection, the primary cause of death in the early 20th century, had been largely vanquished by antibiotics, improved nutrition, and sanitation. Many vitamins had been isolated and manufactured. Their pivotal role, not only in preventing the classical deficiency diseases but also in maintaining optimal health, was gaining increasing recognition.

DNA (deoxyribonucleic acid) had been identified as the carrier of our genetic heredity; scientists were on the brink of determining how genes could be turned on or off to prevent disease. As a high school student, I devoured *The Molecular Biology of the Gene* by James Watson (1965), who was a Nobel Prize winner and one of the scientists credited with discovering the structure of DNA. My mother encouraged my interest by allowing me to bring cages of mice into her basement to perform primitive genetic experiments for the Detroit Metropolitan High School Science Fair.

As a budding young scientist, I was thrilled to be entering medical research at a time of such great promise. Over the next several decades, I became increasingly frustrated as the Amendments thwarted innovation that could have saved millions of lives. Instead of a Golden Age of Health, we ended up with needless premature death, disease, and disability.

Unfortunately, the increased regulations recommended by drug company critics to address their concerns (e.g., soaring drug prices, dwindling innovation, more "me-too" drugs, "excessive" profits, and focus on long-term treatment rather than short-term cures) would serve only to make a bad situation worse. However, we can correct the problems created by the Amendments when we understand how they have distorted the pharmaceutical industry, affected the practice of medicine, and shifted our health care paradigm from prevention to treatment. Only then can we hope to regain the Golden Age of Health that should have already been ours.

Until now, only pharmaceutical industry insiders, a few knowledgeable economists, and those interested in prevention had much reason to suspect that the regulations were so deadly. Each group has only a partial picture of what the Amendments have done.

Throughout my life, I have emphasized prevention, have worked in the pharmaceutical industry, have consulted with nutraceutical (vitamin and supplement) firms, and have familiarized myself with economic principles. Thus, my perspective is more integrated than that of my peers. To explain the negative impact of the Amendments, this book will first address their impact on the pharmaceutical industry, where most of the economic research has been done. This knowledge is necessary for readers to understand the devastating consequences that the Amendments have had on the practice of medicine and how the Amendments shifted us from a prevention-based paradigm to a treatment-based one.

You may be asking yourself, "If the Amendments have had such a dire impact, why haven't I heard about it before?" Without insider information about how the Amendments act behind the scenes, even a dedicated journalist would have a difficult time putting the story together. In addition, most insiders have good reasons to be silent. Blowing the whistle on the Amendments would make their job difficult and might even endanger the financial solvency of their company. Still, many might speak out if they thought their comments would be taken seriously instead of simply being ridiculed. However, if drug companies or their employees tell the American public that the regulations, which were meant to police the pharmaceutical industry and protect consumers, often do just the opposite, then their concerns are likely to be discounted. Such comments would, at best, be labeled politically incorrect and, at worst, self-serving. Why risk your job, your company, and your good name when no one is likely to believe you anyway?

People think the FDA is protecting them—it isn't. What the FDA is doing and what people think it's doing are as different as night and day.
—Dr. Herbert Ley, Commissioner of the FDA, 1968–69

I understand their dilemma. After receiving a BS in biochemistry and a PhD in biophysics from Michigan State University, I did my postdoctoral work at St. Louis University's Department of Surgery and went on to become an assistant professor there. I left in 1976 to join The Upjohn Company, where I remained for 19 years. My job was to discover and develop new drugs, some of which were natural products or chemical modifications. Like many of my colleagues, I had a good idea of why drug prices were on the rise. When I hinted at the deadly secret of the Amendments to people outside the industry, I was met with considerable skepticism.

Today, the situation has greatly changed. In the past few years, new research about the pharmaceutical, medical, and supplement industries has surfaced, which makes it possible to estimate the cost—in lives and money—of the 1962 Amendments in a compelling way. The research detailed in this book is shocking: conservative estimates show that each of us has loved ones whose lives have been shortened by the Amendments (Chapter 27). Our own lives are also at risk.

In addition, the Amendments have empowered uncaring bureaucrats, greedy pharmaceutical executives, charlatans selling questionable supplements, and politicians who will do anything to be reelected, while they have marginalized their ethical, concerned, and honest counterparts (Chapter 20). Terminally ill patients who become of aware of potentially lifesaving treatments tied up in regulatory red tape must turn to the black market or beg for permission—usually unsuccessfully—for a chance to save their lives (Chapters 8).

As a result, the Amendments have sabotaged the Golden Age of Health that awaited us in the 1960s and beyond. Armed with that understanding, we can reverse this tragedy and finally claim our Golden Age of Health.

I invite you to consider the following chapters carefully. The life you save may be your own.

The Thalidomide Tragedy Created an Even Bigger One

I n the 1960s, most people believed—as my family did—that the Amendments were designed to make sure that the United States would never experience a thalidomide tragedy. The Amendments weren't written to protect us against future drug tragedies. They languished in Congress for several years before thalidomide became the biggest drug disaster of its time. The Amendments were never designed to make drugs safer; indeed, they were intended to do something else entirely.

Senator Estes Kefauver introduced the first version of the Amendments in 1960 (Grow 1997, 4), shortly after his 1959 hearings about the drug industry (Temin 1980, 122). The senator believed that consumers wasted their money when they bought more expensive brand-name drugs instead of generics. He felt that his legislation would make it easier for physicians and their patients to trust generic drugs.

In the 1960s, generic drugs weren't as popular as they are today. Although the active ingredients might be chemically identical in both brand-name and generic drugs, the particle sizes in the tablet or capsule might not be the same. The branded capsule or tablet had other ingredients to aid in stability or absorption, which the generic product might not have. Those small differences sometimes produced large changes in how much of a drug entered the bloodstream and how fast it did so. For some patients, such differences could be critical ones (Temin 1980, 122; Jondrow 1972, 87–88). Consequently, physicians were hesitant to prescribe generics.

Senator Kefauver believed that all drugs, including generic ones, must rigorously demonstrate effectiveness before they are marketed. If effectiveness were the ultimate yardstick of quality, people would have greater faith in the less-expensive generics. The senator didn't realize how costly such tests might be and how they would drive up the prices of generic drugs.

Usually, when a pharmaceutical company first introduced an innovative new drug, physicians rushed to prescribe it, especially if the reputation of the pharmaceutical firm was high. Companies strove to associate their name, or brand, with quality so consumers could buy with confidence and doctors would prescribe their drugs. A company's reputation was a much more important factor than it is today. Indeed, a trusted brand name was crucial. Doctors were more likely to prescribe drugs from companies with a good safety record.

Careful manufacturers wooed the public and linked their brand name with safety. Their advertising claimed, for example, that "We have never yet had reported a case of sudden death following the use of our Antitoxin." Others pointed out that their products had been tested and approved by various outside, third-party laboratories (Young 1987, 16).

Brand-name loyalty rewarded the drug manufacturer (company) that always gave the customer what was promised. With a few exceptions, manufacturers reaped what they sowed. Producers of questionable products simply had too few customers to stay in business (Dowling 1968, 124; Wardell & Lasagna 1975, 13).

If the drug proved to be a good seller, smaller companies often copied the drug formula and sold it as a generic rather than a branded drug. The generic drug could be sold at a lower price than a brand-name pharmaceutical, because the cost of copying a drug was much less than the cost of discovering it, testing it, and going through the FDA drug-approval process. However, the generics often didn't perform as well as their brand-name counterparts for the reasons described earlier.

Before passage of the Amendments, the FDA approved drugs that were "safe for their intended use." Manufacturers gave drugs to trusted physicians to test in patients and used the feedback they received to decide if their drug did what it was intended to do. As subsequent studies demonstrated, pharmaceutical firms hesitated to take an ineffective drug to market for fear it would sell poorly or impact negatively on the company's brand (Chapter 31). However, demonstration of effectiveness wasn't legally required for FDA approval.

While Senator Kefauver was unsuccessfully pushing his regulatory changes in Congress, Europe was experiencing the century's worst drug tragedy. Thalidomide had been introduced there as a new, safer sleeping pill. Unlike barbiturates, which were responsible for many suicides and accidental overdoses, thalidomide appeared to have a wide margin of safety—at least for adults (Squires 1989, Z09).

As women began taking thalidomide, they noticed that it also decreased their morning sickness. Consequently, physicians began recommending thalidomide to pregnant women, as did the manufacturer.

Although thalidomide had relatively few problematic side effects in adults, it inhibited the normal development of arms and legs in unborn babies (phocomelia) if taken between days 20 to 41 of pregnancy (BBC 2014). Often, young women did not even know that they were pregnant when they took thalidomide. Consequently, about 12,000 European babies were born with poorly developed or missing limbs. Some babies, with additional developmental defects, died shortly after birth (Meyler 1966, 43–44).

Richardson-Merrell, working with the German company Chemie Grünenthal (now Grünenthal GmbH) that had made thalidomide, applied for FDA approval in the United States. The FDA examiner in charge of reviewing the thalidomide application, Dr. Frances Kelsey, had been concerned about nerve damage (peripheral neuropathy) and had denied permission for US marketing until further studies could be conducted.

Congress felt that the United States had a close call in avoiding Europe's thalidomide tragedy. Kelsey was honored with an award (Kazman

1991, 31), even though she had delayed its approval because of nerve damage rather than its impact on developing babies. Clearly, the FDA already had enough power to stop a potentially dangerous drug from coming to market.

To address the fears of the American people, Congress passed the 1962 Kefauver-Harris Amendments, a modified version of the Senator's earlier proposals. The Amendments, however, were primarily designed to ensure drug effectiveness, not safety. The Amendments were passed because they were readily available to Congress when the American people wanted reassurance, not because they were the right remedy.

Americans wanted Congress to protect them from unsafe drugs. Unfortunately, drugs powerful enough to save lives will almost certainly have unwanted, even deadly, side effects in some people. To make matters worse, our science is not advanced enough to be able to confidently predict who is at risk.

Instead of recognizing and sharing this uncomfortable truth with the American people, Congress passed the Amendments, which had deadly side effects of their own. It's likely that each one of us—patients, pharmaceutical executives, regulators, and Congress itself—is paying the price.

Chapter 3

The FDA Is Given Carte Blanche

The Amendment greatly changed the process of taking a drug from the laboratory bench to the marketplace; a full decade would pass before the new regulatory pattern was established. Perhaps the most-pivotal aspects of the Amendments were the effectiveness provisions.

One of the first things that the FDA attempted to do after passage of the Amendments was to determine if the 4,000+ drugs (Temin 1980, 128) that were already on the market had the "substantial evidence" of effectiveness. The FDA asked the National Academy of Sciences to undertake this gigantic task, which it did from 1966 through 1969 (National Research Council [NRC] 1969).

Thirty panels, each consisting of six doctors, examined drugs from their respective specialties. They considered the public information put out by the manufacturers, the medical literature, and their own experience. Panels could request additional information from the pharmaceutical companies but rarely did (Temin 1980, 133).

The FDA had instructed the panels to rate drugs as "ineffective," "possibly effective," "probably effective," or "effective" for each "indication" or medical problem for which they were sold (NRC 1969, 7). On their own initiative, the National Academy panels added a controversial category, not explicitly requested by the FDA. Termed "ineffective as a fixed combination," this designation referred to medications containing two or more drugs, usually antibiotics. About 40% of the top 200 drugs at the time were such combinations (NRC 1969, 876). The National Academy considered the drugs ineffective if the combination of two or more didn't perform better than the same drugs when taken together but in separate capsules or tablets.

The National Academy's new category represented one side of an ongoing scientific controversy. Some physicians felt that having antibiotic combinations on the market tempted doctors to prescribe them before knowing which of the components was actually effective against the patient's infection. Moreover, giving two antibiotics instead of one would be expected to increase the number of side effects, clearly a detriment to the patient if only one component of the combination was actually needed.

Conversely, in situations where the combination was warranted, patients were more likely to take a single pill faithfully than two pills from separate prescription bottles. The combinations were about 60% less expensive than buying the separate antibiotics, so they saved the patient money as well (Jondrow 1972, 70).

In a life-threatening situation when the sensitivity of the infectious agent to a particular antibiotic was not known or would take too long to determine, giving a combination could make the difference between life and death. For example, if the wrong antibiotic was prescribed, the patient might be too ill to recover by the time a second, more effective one was given. Sometimes giving a combination antibiotic saved lives that would otherwise have been lost.

Combinations had another advantage that wasn't fully appreciated in the 1960s. Bacteria more easily gain resistance to multiple antibiotics when they are given sequentially, rather than together. If your doctor isn't sure which antibiotic you need and prescribes you the wrong one instead of a combination, the bacteria invading your body may develop resistance to both antibiotics taken in sequence. Because it is much harder for bacteria to develop resistance to multiple antibiotics given together, a combination antibiotic may prevent the development of resistance altogether.

Inhibiting antibiotic resistance can be especially important in patients who are susceptible to re-infection, such as the elderly, those with compromised immune systems, or hospitalized patients with other diseases. Such patients are particularly vulnerable. Indeed, combination therapy is now the standard of care for the infectious disease known as AIDS (acquired immune deficiency syndrome). Just as in bacteria, giving a combination of drugs makes it much harder for HIV (human immunodeficiency virus) to develop resistance. Consequently, AIDS is no longer a death sentence.

Bacterial resistance to antibiotics is a serious problem today. Infections by superbugs that are resistant to all known antibiotics have become a life-threatening possibility in virtually every hospital (Zandonella 2013). Indeed, in the 1950s, hospitals were already using combination antibiotics as part of the fight to keep bacteria from developing resistance and turning into superbugs (Barber, Dutton, Beard, et al. 1960, 11–17).

Would resistant microbes be less of a problem today if combination antibiotics had remained on the market? We'll never know, because the National Academy's Drug Efficacy Study recommended their removal, and the FDA concurred. If doctors wanted patients to have two antibiotics at one time, they would have to write two prescriptions, and patients would have to take twice as many pills at a much greater cost. In addition, the FDA's removal of combination antibiotics from the market gave doctors the impression that prescribing multiple antibiotics simultaneously might expose the doctors to accusations of malpractice. By banning combination antibiotics, the FDA altered the practice of medicine.

For some manufacturers, fixed-dose antibiotic combinations contributed substantially to their bottom line. Panalba, a tetracycline and novobiacin combination, first marketed in 1957, accounted for about 13% of Upjohn's sales (Mintz 1969, 875–81). Upjohn sued the FDA in 1969 for the right to an evidentiary hearing so it could question the panel that had recommended Panalba's withdrawal, could address the panel's concerns, and could share emerging data that might influence the FDA's final decision.

However, the FDA refused to allow this hearing on the grounds that Upjohn had to provide substantial evidence of effectiveness first. Upjohn argued that 12 years of commercial success, during which time the FDA had raised no safety questions, *was* substantial evidence that the product was accepted as safe by the FDA and as effective by the medical community (Temin 1980, 133–35).

The FDA did not consider the prescribing behavior of doctors relevant, even though it had relied on a panel of physicians to decide that combination drugs were "ineffective in fixed combinations." In September 1969, the FDA issued new regulations defining substantial evidence as "adequate and well-controlled studies" (Federal Register 1969). A few months later, the US District Court for Delaware ruled that Upjohn's 54 documents in support of Panalba's effectiveness did not meet these new criteria (US District Court of Delaware 1970).

Ironically, few, if any, of the drugs that the FDA left on the market met the new criteria either. The National Academy used clinical experience, not "adequate and well-controlled studies" in its evaluation to grandfather in some drugs, while withdrawing Panalba, other combination drugs, and those considered ineffective.

Both Upjohn and the Pharmaceutical Manufacturers' Association (PMA) pointed out to the court that until the FDA defined its standard of effectiveness in September 1969, clinical experience—not controlled trials—had been acceptable evidence. The Amendments had changed the rules. The PMA argued that Upjohn and other companies should be given time to do the newly required studies and to provide evidence of the utility of antibiotic combinations (Parfet 1969, 1354). Evidence that bacteria were less likely to develop resistance to the combination antibiotics would have been important to consider (Vavra 1967, 801–05; Barber, Dutton, Beard, et al. 1960).

The medical community itself was concerned about losing its right to prescribe. The FDA received fewer than a dozen letters in support of removing Panalba from the market. When Upjohn asked busy doctors to protest the FDA's action, an astounding 3,500 did so (Mintz 1969).

The court ruled against Upjohn in January 1970. In 1973, legal challenges by other firms reached the Supreme Court, which decided that the FDA would be paralyzed if it had to hold hearings for disallowed drugs or to fight in court to have its decisions upheld (Temin 1980, 136–37). Basically, the courts legitimized the FDA's prerogative to remove drugs from the market with as much or as little input from the manufacturer as it desired. The pharmaceutical companies would have virtually no legal recourse, regardless of the merit or capriciousness of the FDA's decision. Companies could be deprived of significant income without due process. When I joined the Upjohn Company in the mid-1970s, it was still reeling from the staggering implications of that decision.

By April 1971, drugs representing about 10% of annual pharmaceutical sales had been rated as "ineffective," "possibly effective," or "ineffective as a fixed combination." The FDA either removed those products from the market or gave manufacturers 6 months to provide data according to the new definition of substantial evidence of effectiveness. Some drugs from the "probably effective" category were also included.

Critics pointed out that 6 months was barely enough time to line up investigators, let alone do the longer and more complex studies that the FDA now wanted (Jondrow 1972, 109–10). In the 1970s, about 7 years were required to perform the human studies (DiMasi 2001a, 286–96), including the human safety trials that the FDA required before effectiveness studies could be performed. The courts were asking the drug companies to perform those studies in a fraction of the required time.

Industry management at this time consisted largely of scientists who had been promoted because of their prowess in the laboratory. They were not savvy politically, had limited business background, and were unprepared for the power tactics wielded by post-Amendment regulators. Consequently, the scientist managers began to be marginalized and were replaced by business executives ready to "fight fire with fire."

Chapter 4

A Revolving Door Swings between Drug Companies and the FDA

The inability to appeal its rulings gave the FDA unprecedented power to determine which companies would prosper and which would not. In most cases, multiple manufacturers have different forms of the next breakthrough drug in their pipeline. The drug that makes it to the market first is usually many times more profitable than the second one. By demanding more studies of one company's drug but not the other, the FDA now had the power to decide which company would reap lucrative first-to-the market profits.

Once a drug company decides to develop a drug, it will spend 12–14 years on average doing the required regulatory studies (Chapter 6). Other companies will likely be developing similar drugs at the same time. Usually, the company that gets the FDA to approve its drug first will establish itself as the market leader. The second company to gain approval will get only a small share of that market—in the neighborhood of 5–10%. Obviously, the company that gains the earliest approval for its entrant in a new drug class will be a big winner compared to its competitors.

If an FDA employee feels negatively toward a company or the personnel representing it, he or she can punish the offending party by simply taking longer to give the go-ahead on the dozens of decision points along the development process. Some companies have even been faced with delayed new drug approvals because of manufacturing violations concerning an already marketed product (Burton 2002; Petersen & Abelson 2002).

> *... Companies are justly fearful of reprisals. Retribution by a regulator can result in the delay of an approval by months or even years and the loss of hundreds and millions of dollars.*
> —Dr. Henry I. Miller, founding director of the FDA's Office of Biotechnology

Naturally, when a regulatory agency can determine which companies win the race to gain approval, the stage is set for corruption. Indeed, in the late 1980s, three generic pharmaceutical firms—Mylan, Barre-National, and Barr Laboratories—hired private investigators who confirmed their suspicions that FDA examiners were taking bribes to favor their competitors (Higgs 1994; New York Times 1989; Kolberg 1987). The chief executive of Barr Laboratories later complained that the FDA retaliated against that company for this exposé by further delaying its approvals and increasing the frequency of its regulatory inspections (Brimelow & Spencer 1993, 116).

The FDA dragged its feet on Barr's generic drug applications even beyond the time that the agency was legally required to rule on them. Because the FDA had actually violated the law, Barr sued. The FDA blamed the "Generic Drug Scandal," uncovered by the three firms, for causing the agency to lose employees and for slowing its application processing. In other words, because FDA employees had accepted bribes and been fired, generic companies—and specifically the whistleblowers—must now suffer delays for the sins of the regulators.

The US Court of Appeals, District of Columbia Circuit, acknowledged that the FDA had violated the law. Instead of insisting that the FDA review Barr's applications, however, the court concluded that doing so would give Barr an unfair advantage over its competitors, who had suffered similar delays without initiating suit (US Court 1991). The FDA was not instructed to stop breaking the law; the drug companies were essentially told that the courts would let them be punished for complaining about it.

> *When asked why they do not protest against unreasonable delays or demands, pharmaceutical leaders usually offer the reason that there are implicit or explicit threats of punitive or retaliatory action by the FDA if the drug houses elect to fight.*
> —Louis Lasagna, founder of the Tufts Center for the Study of Drug Development

Such court rulings from the late 1960s to early 1990s essentially told the pharmaceutical industry that the FDA had carte blanche in dealing with them. Even when the FDA did not meet its legal obligations, companies could expect no relief.

> *The FDA is standing there with a machine gun against the pharmaceutical industry, so you better be their friend rather than their enemy. They are the boss. If you're a pharmaceutical firm, they own you body and soul.*
> —G. Kirk Raab, Genetech CEO, 1990–95

In dealing with FDA regulators, I usually found them to be sincere individuals who are trying to protect the American public. However, power corrupts and sets the stage for abuse. FDA employees are only human and respond to incentives. If company representatives rub them the wrong way, regulators avoid dealing with those individuals by putting their applications at the back of the queue. If an FDA examiner actively dislikes (and therefore distrusts) someone from industry, the review process is likely to go forward more slowly. When pharmaceutical executives deal with the FDA, they have to tread carefully or risk—quite literally—years of retaliation.

> *… 84% of companies polled in 1991 reported declining to file a complaint against the FDA for fear of retaliation.*
> —Peter Brimelow and Leslie Spencer, **Forbes**, 1993

In self-defense, pharmaceutical companies began hiring former FDA employees to successfully navigate the agency's culture rather than relying on a scientist-manager whose skill set might not include politically correct speech and the deference that regulators expected.

If those people at the FDA didn't like you, you were dead, and if they did like you, it didn't make any difference what kind of crap was in your application.
—David W. Nelson, chief investigator for Representative John Dingell about FDA and drug companies

Critics of the pharmaceutical industry decry this practice as a revolving door between the FDA and drug companies. In reality, hiring regulators who help interface with the FDA has been a necessary survival tactic created by the Amendments.

Before the Amendments passed, 10% of FDA officials leaving the agency from 1959 to 1963 went into the pharmaceutical industry (Garrison 1970, 75). By 1969, that percentage had increased to an incredible 76% (Lynes 1989, 22). After the Amendments passed, more than seven times as many regulators left the FDA to join drug companies than before. Indeed, most left the agency primarily to guide those firms through the ever-expanding regulatory labyrinth.

Former regulators can advise a company about the agency's mindset and can help ensure fewer misunderstandings and conflicts. Their network at the FDA allows them to alert the company at an early stage whether or not certain types of drugs will receive favorable treatment by the FDA.

When interactions between the FDA and drug companies become strained, the ultimate loser isn't only the drug company. Terminally ill patients, some of them children, never get access to lifesaving medications.

For example, an immune booster, mifamurtide, was found to reduce the risk of death by 28% when given to young osteosarcoma patients along with standard chemotherapy (Mepact n.d.). Osteosarcoma is a rare cancer affecting mostly children and young adults, with under 1,000 new US cases per year.

In 2009, mifamurtide was approved for use in the European Union as well as in Iceland, Norway, and Liechtenstein. The United Kingdom approved it in 2011. Mifamurtide, coupled with chemotherapy, is now the standard of care in those countries for children with osteosarcoma. One of the drug's champions, Dr. Paul Meyers at Memorial Sloan Kettering Cancer Center in New York, says his goal is to get the drug approved in 194 of the 195 countries on earth.

The country that Meyers has little hope for is the United States. The FDA has been refusing to approve it since 2007.

Like many breakthrough drugs, mifamurtide had many setbacks. Because osteosarcoma was an orphan disease with small numbers of patients, Ciba Geigy decided to stop making it in the middle of a pivotal Phase 3 trial. Jenner Therapeutics picked up the drug and made enough of it to finish the study before going out of business. IDM Pharma bought Jenner's assets, including mifamurtide.

Although the Phase 3 trial had been completed, the survival data had never been examined. When IDM Pharma scientists analyzed it, they contacted Meyers to tell him the good news: mifamurtide, added to standard chemotherapy, kept the osteosarcoma patients alive better than chemotherapy alone. The drug worked!

"We went to the FDA [with these new results]," Meyers explained, "and we had an extraordinarily hostile reception. I mean a really nasty, angry, 'Get out of my face, what the hell are you doing here' reception." He speculates that the FDA was upset that he and his colleague didn't discuss the design of their study with the regulators before undertaking it—as would be commonly done by pharmaceutical firms. Drug companies hire former FDA regulators to interface with the agency to ensure that they are aware of such unstated expectations.

Even after the European Union had approved mifamurtide and a Japanese company, Takeda, acquired it, the FDA refused to look at the survival data. Instead, the agency demanded another trial with about 900 patients, roughly the number of patients diagnosed with osteosarcoma in the United States each year. Because of the small number of patients who would use this drug, Takeda couldn't justify the extra cost and didn't undertake development.

To add insult to injury, the FDA stopped "compassionate use" of the drug in 2012. This program, which allows a few select patients to try a new drug before it's approved, will be described in later chapters. As a result of the FDA's action, however, Americans now have no legal access to mifamurtide. Those who want the best treatment for their children with osteosarcoma must go overseas for almost a year to get the therapy—even though it was first discovered and proven effective in the United States (Olsen 2015, 61–82). Needless to say, few families can afford the costs of treatment and a year overseas, so mifamurtide is unavailable to most US children who need it to stay alive.

> *After my testimony, a number of drug-company employees came up and thanked me for saying what they couldn't say. Some told me that they wanted to applaud but didn't dare. However, one drug-company employee approached me, looking pale and drawn, with his company's chief lawyer beside him. He expressed his anger at me for quoting his criticisms of the FDA in my testimony.... He explained that their company had a major new drug up for approval with the FDA and that the agency could delay its approval and cost his company a lot of money.*
> —David R. Henderson, Research Fellow with the Hoover Institution at Stanford University describing his congressional testimony

Offending the FDA is not just a blow to a drug company's bottom line. It's deadly for those who need a lifesaving drug that doesn't make it to the US market.

Because of the FDA's ability and willingness to retaliate against those who do not do things the agency's preferred way, this book would not be possible if I were still employed by a pharmaceutical firm. After I left the Upjohn Company, I presented some of this book's material at scientific conventions (Ruwart 2004). Researchers from numerous companies congratulated me on speaking out. They also told me that they wouldn't dare to do the same for fear of retaliation by the FDA against their employer.

I've shared a bit of this information with FDA personnel and received sympathetic feedback (Ruwart 2005a). However, some regulators would likely feel attacked and slow down the approvals of my employer, if I had one, thereby putting the entire company at risk.

Now you know why you haven't heard this story before. Only a few older insiders are truly aware of how the Amendments have reshaped the pharmaceutical industry, negatively impacted the practice of medicine, and shifted our healing paradigm from disease prevention to treatment after the fact.

Chapter 5

Is "Safe and Effective" a Myth?

A s the Panalba example illustrates, "effectiveness" does not mean the same thing to everyone. The Drug Efficacy Study's category of "ineffective in fixed combinations" shows how diverse the meaning of drug effectiveness really is. Let's take a look at some other examples.

Does a drug need to work for half of the patients who take it, or does it need to work for each one? If the drug works for only 10% of the patients who will be treated with it, is it effective enough to be marketed? Does it make a difference if they are totally cured of a disease that would otherwise kill them?

Consider an anti-cancer drug. If it slows down cancer growth so that most people live a few weeks longer, is that drug "effective"? If the drug cures 10% of those who take it but simply wastes the money of the other 90%, should it be approved?

The definition of "effective," at least as it applies to pharmaceuticals, is not obvious. In 1911, the Supreme Court was asked to rule whether names of drugs and patent medicines that implied or claimed a curative effect were fraudulent. The Court ruled that "a claim that certain beneficial results will follow the use of a prescribed drug or medicine obviously is not a statement of an existing fact, but is a forecast concerning a future event and is in the nature of things *an expression of an opinion*" [emphasis mine] (US Supreme Court 1911).

Because of our genetic diversity and the impact of environmental factors, no drug works for everyone. One benefit of having several me-too drugs on the market is that the small differences in chemical structure can mean big differences in how an individual's body reacts. Thus, if one blood pressure medication does not effectively treat your hypertension or gives you undesirable side effects, your doctor may switch you to a similar medication with better success.

The well-documented placebo effect adds further confusion to the definition of effectiveness. When people are given a sugar pill, many respond as if they had been given an effective drug for such diverse conditions as pain, depression, Parkinson's disease, irritable bowel syndrome, cancer, etc. The magnitude of the placebo effect varies with circumstances (Price, Finniss, & Benedetti 2008, 565–90) such as conscious beliefs of the patient, subconscious conditioning, and even genetics (Furmark, Appel, Henningsson, et al. 2008, 13066–743). The ways in which placebos work are still poorly understood. Although no drug is effective in everyone, every drug will likely be effective in some people as a result of the placebo effect. Consequently, one could argue that there is no such thing as an ineffective drug.

... the FDA definition of effectiveness as "effective beyond a placebo" is an improper policy that is detrimental to public health. The effectiveness standards deny consumers the benefit of a proven placebo treatment that would improve their condition, even when this may be the only, or at least the safest, treatment available.
—Russell S. Sobel, professor of Economics and Entrepreneurship,
The Citadel, Charleston, SC

We face similar problems in deciding if a drug is safe. The Amendments weren't designed to improve safety, even though they were passed to reassure an American public concerned about having a thalido-mide-like tragedy in the United States.

The Amendments probably couldn't have prevented the thalidomide tragedy in Europe, even if they had been part of the regulatory landscape there. In the early 1960s, the sensitivity of the unborn baby to drugs that were well tolerated by the mother was not widely appreciated (Heaton 1994, 40), so the manufacturer did no additional testing when it began recommending the drug for morning sickness.

Moreover, even if such testing had been undertaken, thalidomide's devastating impact on the unborn probably would not have been seen. Small laboratory animals can't take pills, so drugs must be given in a solution. Thalidomide degrades if the solution isn't acidic enough, but this fact wasn't understood by some researchers attempting to reproduce what happened in humans in the early 1960s (Schardein 1976, 5).

Consequently, animal tests at first suggested that thalidomide harmed only the offspring of rabbits and monkeys (Schardein 1976), even though researchers eventually found that most mammals were affected (Botting 2015, 183–98). Today, because of what we learned from thalidomide, we test drugs in pregnant animals in the hopes that any problems will show up in the laboratory rather than in our children.

However, we can never be sure that what we see (or don't see) in animals will be seen (or not seen) in people. Only about half of the side effects that will occur in humans show up in animal tests. About one-fifth of the side effects seen in animals never even happen in people (Litchfield 1962, 665–72). Animal testing improves the odds of knowing what problems a new drug may have, but it's hardly a sure thing.

Even the limited human studies that are done before a drug is marketed cannot always predict what side effects will be seen with widespread use. People are very different genetically, so some will suffer side effects that other people won't experience. Variations in diet, nutrition, and environmental conditions also influence who can take a drug safely and who cannot.

Consequently, anyone taking a new drug should be aware that all of its side effects are not known. Testing—even in people—can uncover and predict only so much. Even today—with some notable exceptions that we'll discuss later—most of the serious side effects of marketed drugs usually result from our lack of scientific knowledge, not from manufacturer negligence.

No amount of regulation or testing will uncover every problem that a drug has. Because the risk of side effects is always present, we must use caution when taking drugs. Drugs are powerful substances, which is why they can heal. However, that same power can harm as well.

Unfortunately, the American public has been conditioned to believe that FDA approval is equivalent to a guarantee of both safety and effectiveness. Putting the words "safe and effective" in the FDA's search engine shows that this terminology is used throughout the website (e.g., "Development of Safe and Effective Tumor Vaccines and Gene Therapy Products") (see also Puri n.d.). Clearly, this language creates an expectation that the consumer can rely on FDA-approved products to be exactly that: safe and effective.

Ironically, if a pharmaceutical manufacturer advertised that its FDA-approved drug was safe and effective, it is highly likely that the FDA would censure the company. Ads you see on television for prescription drugs always have a long list of cautions and side effects because the FDA insists on it.

As regulators, physicians, and industry insiders know, there is no such thing as a drug that can be counted on to be safe and effective in everyone. Even lifesaving drugs, such as penicillin, kill people every year from allergic or other idiosyncratic (poorly understood) side effects. People die every year from gastrointestinal bleeding caused by seemingly innocuous aspirin, sold without a prescription.

Because no drug is totally safe and effective, no drug is worthy of FDA approval if the standard is safety and effectiveness. Put another way, if the FDA approved only drugs that were totally safe and effective, we would have no new drugs at all.

Wisely, the FDA has decided to use a risk-to-benefit assessment, rather than insist on total safety and efficacy (effectiveness) for new drug approvals. However, this yardstick is clearly subjective because the risk-to-benefit ratio cannot be calculated systematically with so much person-to-person variability.

Chapter 6

The FDA Becomes
the Scapegoat

B ecause no drug is totally safe and effective, FDA personnel risk censure by Congress whenever the unexpected side effects, which occur with all drugs, are severe enough to attract public attention. The Amendments made this problem worse.

Before passage of the Amendments, approval was automatic if the FDA didn't object to the drug company's application to market a new drug in the following 6 months. The Amendments, however, required FDA officials to sign off on an approval, thereby putting their heads in the proverbial noose.

Clearly, the regulators became concerned by the new visibility that the 1962 Amendments had given them. They were asked to approve only safe and effective drugs, a clearly impossible task. To protect themselves, regulators demanded that the pharmaceutical firms do more testing so that the regulators could show Congress that they had done their "due diligence" if the FDA had to defend its approval of a particular drug. Requiring more studies was easy because the Supreme Court had ruled that the FDA's decisions could not be challenged by the pharmaceutical firms.

The Amendments, coupled with the Supreme Court's ruling, gave the agency unprecedented power over every aspect of pharmaceutical development: which animal studies needed to be done before human testing,

Figure 1. Average Development Time of New Chemical Entities before (black bars)[1] and after (gray bars)[2] Passage of the 1962 Kefauver-Harris Amendments.[3]

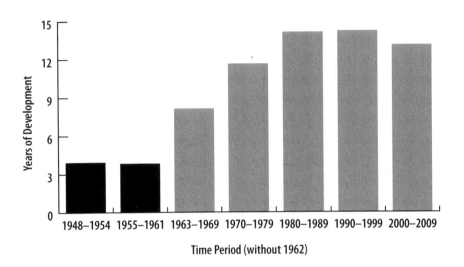

how clinical trials were designed and how many people were tested, how the drug was to be manufactured, what recordkeeping was needed, and even (in possible violation of the First Amendment to the US Constitution) what companies could tell doctors and patients about their drugs. This power was open-ended, thereby allowing the FDA to keep increasing the requirements that new drugs had to meet year after year. Pharmaceutical companies dared not protest for fear that the FDA would drag its feet when reviewing their New Drug Applications (NDAs).

Of course, meeting all of the new requirements took time. As shown in Figure 1, the estimated development times for new drugs (i.e., the length of time between discovering or making a new drug and taking it to the market) were about 4 years between 1948 and 1961. From 1963 to 1969, development times soared to more than 8 years and rose to more than 14 years in the following decades.

By 1992, FDA review time for new drugs averaged 31.3 months (Cantor 1997). In that year, the Prescription Drug User Fee Act (PD-UFA) (Kaitin 2003, 357–71), which we'll discuss further in Chapter 31, was passed to give the FDA more funds to hire reviewers. The 13-month decrease in development time shown in Figure 1 for 2000–09 new drug approvals was primarily caused by PDUFA's reduction in the time required for the FDA to review the NDA.

The term "new drug" in this book refers to "new chemical entities," or NCEs. An NCE is an entirely new drug rather than just a change in the amount of drug per pill or a dosage type (capsule or tablet, for example). In recent years, we've started using the term "new molecular entities," or NMEs, instead of NCEs because some new drugs aren't "chemicals" but "biological products," such as cloned antibodies and small proteins. NCEs and NMEs do not include vaccines.

The FDA doesn't perform the required studies themselves; the pharmaceutical firms must execute them. By the time I left the industry in 1995, an NDA, which included the results of such studies, filled—quite literally—an entire truckload with paper. The FDA reviewed this paperwork and rejected the new drug, asked for more studies, or approved the new drug for marketing.

As you might imagine, the FDA needed a great deal of time to look through all the data, although much had already been reviewed so that the FDA could advise the company what was needed at various steps along the way. The Amendments required the FDA to limit its review time of NDAs to 6 months (Kaplan 1995, 179–96, esp. 195). Instead, review time went from about 7 months pre-Amendment to an average of 29 months between 1963 and 1969. More than half of the increase in development time during this period was due to the increase in FDA's review time. Even though the FDA wasn't meeting its legal mandate, the drug companies dared not complain.

In the early 1980s, when the average review time was 2.5 years, Dr. Henry Miller, who headed the review team for recombinant human insulin, recommended its approval after a mere 4 months of review. Humulin, as the drug would be called, was truly a breakthrough for diabetics. Until that time, insulin was derived from animal sources. With long-term use, 10–50% of diabetics developed allergic reactions, some of which could be life-threatening. Humulin and its successors would reduce allergic reactions to 3% or less (Idlebrook 2014).

However, Miller's supervisor didn't want to act on the recommendation, even though the supervisor agreed with it. He was afraid that Congress and other FDA critics would accuse him of acting with undue haste if the product didn't perform as expected. Luckily for US diabetics, when his supervisor went on vacation, Miller (2000, 41–42) was able to convince his supervisor's boss to sign off on the approval.

The Amendments created a disincentive for regulators to approve new drugs by forcing FDA officials to sign off on new drug approvals. Regulators did so only by putting their own jobs at risk should anything go wrong.

Chapter 7

AIDS Patients Take Matters into Their Own Hands

T he terminally ill can't wait 14 years or so for lifesaving treatments to make it through the system. When US AIDS victims discovered that other countries—with fewer regulatory requirements—frequently had more new drugs, they started going overseas to bring home new therapies not yet approved by the FDA (e.g., ribavirin [Roberts, Dickinson, Heseltine, et al. 1990, 884–92) and Isoprinosine (Pedersen, Sandstrom, Petersen, et al. 1990, 1757–63). Sometimes when AIDS victims returned, US customs agents confiscated their new hope at the border.

The resulting protests by the AIDS community persuaded then–FDA Commissioner Frank Young to allow importation of small quantities of medications that were marketed in other countries for individual use (*Wall Street Journal* 1988, 39). Young's successors did not always share his compassion and sporadically ordered the seizure of imported pharmaceuticals (Life Extension Foundation 1995, 1–5).

We're not prepared to march into people's homes like the Gestapo and take drugs away from desperately ill people.
—Dr. Frank Young, former FDA commissioner (1984–89)

When the AIDS epidemic began, several scientists (myself included) started working on potential treatments. The scientific community, even in drug companies, is not very secretive. AIDS Buyers Clubs quickly identified which new drugs were undergoing development and then hired chemists to make them for distribution throughout the AIDS community (Kolata 1991, A1; Larson 1992, 48–50; Sherman 1992, 62–69; Kwitny 1992).

One AIDS activist claimed that more bootleg ddC (an anti-AIDS drug in the early stages of human testing) was distributed through their network than was given to AIDS sufferers enrolled in the FDA-mandated clinical studies (US FDA 1991). Information from the patients who took ddC and their doctors could have been invaluable in assisting in drug development. However, the illegality of the entire operation made gathering such data difficult. From the reports that are available, the AIDS community apparently had a good system of keeping up with potential side effects and sharing information within its ranks (Kwitny 1992).

The Buyers Clubs violated the pharmaceutical firms' patents for the new drugs, but the companies wisely declined to prosecute their future customers (Kwitny 1992). Clearly, making and selling those potentially lifesaving drugs before FDA approval was against the law, but the FDA often took no action against most violators, especially those in California who were well organized and vocal. Had the FDA been aggressive with the AIDS patients, the public backlash would have been severe when Americans became aware of how long it actually took a lifesaving new drug to jump through the regulatory hoops.

Instead, the FDA selectively prosecuted those who were least likely to fight back. The 2013 award-winning movie, *Dallas Buyers Club*, shows how Texas electrician, Ron Woodroof, an AIDS patient given 30 days to live, set up a Buyers Club. The FDA prosecuted him, possibly because he didn't draw media attention as easily as the California AIDS activists. Ultimately, Woodroof lived about 7 years longer than his doctor had predicted, suggesting that the Buyers Clubs were, at least on occasion, able to extend the lives of their members.

The Buyers Clubs generally acted responsibly. Hoffmann-LaRoche was able to obtain bootleg samples of its own drug, ddC, from the New York and San Francisco Buyers Clubs. At that time, FDA approval was still a half-year away, so the AIDS community was making ddC and distributing it illegally.

In early 1992, the FDA's analysis of the capsules, which were supposed to be 0.25 mg, showed a range of 0% to 230% of the intended dose. Both Buyers Clubs shut down sales and retested their supplies, finding a range of 76% to 160%. The clubs contracted with another supplier to make capsules with better quality control (Kwitny 1992, 423–24).

Chapter 8

Courts Rule We Can't Save Our Lives with Unapproved Drugs

n theory, the FDA can grant a desperately ill patient permission to take a drug that is not yet approved. Such expanded access programs are sometimes known as "compassionate use" or "treatment INDs" (investigational new drugs). However, the FDA does not always grant this expanded access.

In addition, the doctor of the compassionate-use patient must spend about 100 hours filling out the necessary paperwork! Needless to say, few physicians can put in this much time per patient. The FDA claims that it has since simplified its forms (US FDA 2018).

Even when the FDA agrees to expanded access, pharmaceutical companies are often reluctant to give terminal patients a drug that is still in development. If patients die from organ failure related to their disease, the FDA may require additional studies from the manufacturer to make sure that the death was not hurried along by the drug. Naturally, the extra studies increase the development timeline and overall cost.

A more ruthless competitor, who withholds a drug from the desperately ill, won't be burdened with those extra studies. The competitor can pull ahead in the race to the market; the compassionate company can lose its "first-to-the market" status as a result. First-to-market pharmaceuticals in a new class of drugs can capture up to 90% of the marketplace, leaving other drugs of the same class a much smaller slice. This is just one example of how the Amendments empowered those focused on profits and penalized those focused on patients. Compassion is often penalized, sometimes quite heavily.

Consequently, cancer patients often face a great deal of frustration when attempting to get expanded access. In March 2001, Abigail Burroughs, a college student with a squamous cell carcinoma of the head and neck, tried to get access to Erbitux, a drug that specifically targeted Abigail's type of cancer. Erbitux looked promising even in early human studies.

At first, Abigail's father tried to get her into a clinical trial, which was part of the formal testing program required by the FDA. When that approach failed, he appealed to the FDA and his congressional representatives for treatment under the expanded access program. For months, the FDA refused to allow Abigail access to the drug; she finally succumbed to her disease in June 2001 (Kovach 2007).

Frank Burroughs, in honor of his daughter, formed the Abigail Alliance, which brought suit against the FDA on the grounds that the US Constitution protects the right of terminally ill patients to buy drugs not yet FDA approved. The Alliance argued that cancer patients and the terminally ill should be allowed to buy drugs that had been tested in humans for safety (Phase 1) but not for effectiveness. In 2006, the same year that Erbitux was approved and considered a breakthrough drug for squamous cell carcinoma (Vermorken, Mesia, Rivera, et al. 2008, 1116–27), the US Court of Appeals for the District of Columbia ruled in favor of the Abigail Alliance (US Court of Appeals 2006).

The Court of Appeals later re-evaluated its own decision at the request of the FDA. On August 7, 2007, the Court reversed itself, ruling that patients do not have the Constitutional right to attempt to save their lives with drugs that aren't FDA approved (US Court of Appeals 2007). The Alliance appealed to the Supreme Court, which refused to hear the case. The lower court ruling prevailed by default.

Under the Fifth Amendment's guarantee that "No person shall be deprived of life, liberty or property without due process of law," a critically ill patient should have access to a potentially lifesaving drug that has been deemed safe for human consumption, if the patient agrees to bear the risks involved. But earlier this year, the Supreme Court refused to hear a case on the issue, denying countless patients their right to pursue life.

—Gideon J. Sofer, cancer patient, *Wall Street Journal*, December 30, 2008

Consequently, desperate patients with terminal illnesses make unapproved drugs in their kitchen and share the results with others with the same diseases (Marcus 2012). Some dying patients and those with debilitating diseases are going to gain access to new drug therapies; the only question is whether they will get them from a company with good manufacturing practices, the black market, or their own attempts at kitchen chemistry.

Chapter 9

Americans Die Waiting While Brits Enjoy "Made in America" Drugs First

A t the time it happened, the thalidomide tragedy was the largest drug disaster in pharmaceutical history. We might expect that both manufacturers and regulators would do additional testing to prevent a future tragedy. However, the Amendments would prove to be—quite literally—regulatory overkill, especially compared to how other nations reacted.

In some cases, overseas agencies weren't lax; they just did things differently. For example, Britain had already realized that more pre-approval studies probably wouldn't uncover more toxicity because safety problems usually resulted from insufficient know-how. Instead, British regulatory agencies focused on post-approval studies, which monitored what happened when large numbers of people took the drug. If scientific ignorance, rather than carelessness, was the cause of most withdrawals, the Brits hoped to catch the problems soon after approval.

In 1960, the time needed to get a new, self-originated drug from the lab bench to the US marketplace was just slightly longer than in Britain (2.9 vs. 2.5 years, respectively) (LG Thomas 1990, 497–517, esp. 514, Appendix). After the thalidomide incident, Britain passed some new safety measures but didn't implement an effectiveness requirement until 1971 (Grabowski, Vernon, & Thomas 1978, 133–63, esp. 144–45). By 1970, US development times were 10.0 years vs. 4.2 years in Britain (LG Thomas 1990). By 1980, after the British added effectiveness regulations, US development times were still twice as long as Britain's (12.0 vs. 5.8 years) (LG Thomas 1990).

In Britain, development costs rose too but only at half the rate of increase that the United States experienced (Grabowski, Vernon, & Thomas 1978). In other words, even though development times and costs increased in Britain after the thalidomide tragedy, they were still half of what the Amendments imposed on the US drug market. In Chapter 31, we'll examine the negative health impact of this strategy on the Brits.

Before the Amendments, most first-in-human studies with drugs discovered in the United States were done here. By the mid-1970s, fewer than half were (Lasagna & Wardell 1975, 157). When we wanted to develop a new drug, we increasingly started development overseas because we could test it in humans—and market it there—much sooner than the FDA would allow. If the drug worked well in the foreign studies, we began human trials in the United States.

Consequently, in the first couple of decades following the Amendments, about twice as many new drugs were introduced in Britain than in the United States. When a drug was approved in both countries, Britain generally had it years before it was available in the United States. Because many new drugs were for cardiovascular disease, which is the number one killer in the developed world, many Americans who might have had a longer life without the Amendments died prematurely (Wardell 1978, 133–45; Grabowski 1980; US GAO 1980).

One of the new drugs was propranolol, the first beta-blocker for heart disease. Because of the "drug lag" between British and US marketing of this drug, propranolol didn't enter the American market until 1968, 3 years after it had been available in Europe. One study performed in the 1980s estimated that propranolol was saving about 10,000 American lives per year (Arthur D Little Inc. 1984, I). Consequently, the 3-year delay in propranolol approval cost approximately 30,000 Americans lives. This estimate may be low, because propranolol was not approved in the

United States for its major uses—angina and hypertension—until 1973 and 1976, respectively.

Instead of being complemented for finally approving propranolol, a congressional committee criticized the FDA for exposing the American public to a drug with potential safety problems (Lasagna 1989, 322–43; Wardell 1979, 25–33, esp. 30). Because all drugs have side effects, Congress was essentially telling the FDA not to approve any drugs at all. Given this negative feedback, it's hardly surprising that the FDA increased its regulatory demands even further.

In the early 1970s, more than two-thirds of the drugs discovered in the United States and introduced first in Britain weren't even available in the United States. Those drugs that were eventually approved by the FDA came to the United States years behind their British introduction (Grabowski 1980, 5–36).

Some of the drugs lost to the US market—or greatly delayed—were classified as important therapeutic advances by the FDA (Grabowski 1980). The drug lag continued throughout the 1980s, depriving Americans of lifesaving medicine (Kaitin, Mattison, Northington, et al. 1989, 121–38). Delays in approving second-generation beta-blockers and hypertensive agents, which were safer than the first-generation ones, resulted in a number of unnecessary deaths. Few people realized that regulatory delays were responsible (Wardell & Lasagna 1975, 50–77).

… there is a different kind of hazard to public health, posed by the prolonged delays and great costs of developing new and potentially useful drugs which the FDA's own protective systems have imposed. In some respects, the agency has become a formidable roadblock.
—The President's Biomedical Research Panel, Appendix A, US Department of Health, Education, and Welfare, Publication No. OS76-50, 1976

The United States had more anti-cancer drugs in its pharmacies than any other nation had between 1960 and 1975. During the following 15 years, the United States had fewer anti-cancer drugs than did France,

Germany, the United Kingdom (UK), and Japan as a result of what came to be known as the drug lag. In the earlier period, the United States got new anti-cancer drugs about 1.5 years before the UK. In the second period, US introductions lagged behind the UK by about 0.9 years (Kaitin & Brown 1995, 361–73).

A similar pattern emerged with NBEs (new biologically based entities), such as recombinant proteins, vaccines, and monoclonal antibodies. Although 82% of those originated in the United States and began clinical testing there, only 25% of them were first introduced in the United States.

Although 50 psychotropic drugs were marketed in Europe by 1993 and 20 were highly rated by experts, only one of them was in testing in the United States in that year. Because the drugs were close to losing patent protection by the time the FDA would have approved them, most never appeared on US pharmacy shelves (Kaitin & Brown 1995).

Until recently, the FDA required that all studies for US approval be conducted in the United States, so we usually had to repeat what we already had done overseas. Because the FDA regularly wanted more studies than did other drug regulatory agencies, our drugs were often marketed overseas years before the FDA approved them.

As the US pharmaceutical industry put more money into development, it had less to put into innovation. Instead, US firms had to license foreign drug discoveries for their development portfolio. In the mid-1970s, about 25% of the drugs developed by US companies were licensed from foreign firms; by 1982, that number had doubled (Wardell 1982).

Europe still gets many cutting-edge treatments before the United States does. Since 1996, for example, Peptide Receptor Radionuclide Therapy (PRRT) has been available in Europe for treatment of neuroendocrine carcinoma. Steve Jobs, founder and CEO of Apple, was diagnosed with one of those rare cancers in 2004. They are often difficult to detect, to surgically remove, and to destroy.

PRRT uses a drug called octreotide to bind to receptors found primarily on cancer cells. A radioactive compound is attached to the octreotide so that the cancer will be killed by radiation without damaging much of the surrounding tissue. Such treatment has fewer side effects than chemotherapy does, and it slows the cancer's progression for almost 2 years longer than chemotherapy alone. More than 80% of patients benefit (Kwekkeboom, Kam, Van Essen, et al. 2010, R53–73). In spite of this remarkable statistic, this therapy is not available in the United States.

Trials are beginning at the University of Iowa with octreotide minus the radioactivity. The step-by-step process that the FDA demands will delay PRRT's entry into the United States even further. In the meantime, Americans will need to go overseas for treatment that has been available for 20 years in Europe (Olsen 2015, 83–88). Even more depressing, by the time today's PRRT is available in the United States, this therapy will already be obsolete, because second generation versions are already being tested overseas.

Chapter 10

Millions of Americans Die Waiting for Lifesaving Drugs

A s the previous chapter illustrated, the lengthening development times created by the Amendments can have serious side effects of their own. People may die needlessly because the drugs that would extend their lives are still tangled up in regulatory red tape.

Dr. Frank Lichtenberg, a professor at the Columbia University Graduate School of Business and a research associate of the National Bureau of Economic Research, estimated that the NCEs (new chemical entities) approved during 1970–91 saved about 18,800 life-years in 1991 and presumably continued to do so in each subsequent year (Lichtenberg 2003a, 74–109).

It's quite difficult to measure exactly how many lives the average drug saves. For now, we will assume that 18,800 life-years per NCE is about right. Chapter 31 demonstrates that even if Lichtenberg's estimates are too high by a factor of 10 or more, the Amendments will remain—quite literally—regulatory overkill.

Researchers prefer to measure the years of life saved rather than number of the lives saved. A drug that prevents the death of a child, who will live to be 100 years old, for example, will save more life years than a drug that prevents the death of someone who is already 90 years old and will live to be 100.

However, most of us are used to thinking in terms of lives, not life-years. How do we convert life-years to lives in an appropriate manner?

Lichtenberg estimated that new drugs approved between 1970 and 1991 were responsible for about 45% of the decrease in disease-related loss of life during that time (Lichtenberg 2003). Most of those drugs acted on two out of the three major causes of death in the United States: cardiovascular disease (e.g., heart attacks) and cerebrovascular disease (e.g., stroke) (US Census Bureau 2012a, 103, Table 117).

Death rates from heart attacks have plunged more than 50% since 1980 (Xu, Murphy, Kochanek, et al. 2016), while strokes have declined by almost 40% (Medtap International n.d., 4). About half of the decline in deaths resulting from those aliments has been attributed to pharmaceuticals. Lifestyle changes—such as alterations in diet, exercise, and nutrient supplementation, as well as surgical interventions—are believed to be responsible for the rest (Gieringer 1985, 177–201, esp. 185–87; Cutler, McClellan, & Newhouse 1997; Fang, Perraillon, Ghosh, et al. 2014, 608–15; Heidenreich & McClellan 2001, 363–410). The decline in cancer deaths, the third major cause of death in the United States, was not comparable.

Thus, drugs that address heart attacks and stroke were the dominant lifesavers during the years that Lichtenberg studied. The average person saved from heart disease or stroke by drugs gained about 11 years of life (US Census Bureau 1994, 102, Table 138).[4] Thus, new drugs approved during 1970–91 saved about 1,709 lives (18,800 life-years/11 years) annually.

In several of his studies, Lichtenberg discovered that in some years, life expectancy would have gone down without the introduction of new drugs (Lichtenberg 2003). Our American lifestyle—with limited daily exercise, frequent meals of fast food, consumption of excess calories, deficiencies of critical nutrients, and ever-increasing obesity—is compromising our health. Although drugs can alleviate some problems caused by poor lifestyle choices, prevention is ultimately the better alternative. Unfortunately, research in disease prevention has been hampered by the diversion of funds into drug development (Chapter 32).

Because of how the Amendments have suppressed the information flow about inexpensive prevention (Chapters 32–36), many doctors find themselves unable to appropriately counsel their patients in healthy lifestyle choices other than with general recommendations to lose weight and exercise more. As a result, many people choose to take drugs, even with their accompanying side effects, instead of changing the way they live and eat. Of course, some people will have health problems even with lifestyle modifications because of their genetic inheritance. Still others will do poorly because our knowledge about prevention is incomplete.

Heart disease and stroke aren't the only diseases for which regulatory red tape has delayed the availability of lifesaving drugs. In fact, the Abigail Alliance has recommended that FDA approval be granted to 12 cancer drugs years before the FDA allowed them to be marketed. In 2007, the Abigail Alliance calculated that 1,615,200 cancer patients died waiting in the interim. Because many of those drugs would have worked in cancers other than the specific type they were approved for, the number of people who could have benefited might be as high as an additional 4.7 million (Trowbridge & Walker 2007, A17).

Every drug for cancer and other serious life-threatening illnesses that the Abigail Alliance has pushed for earlier access to in our thirteen-year history is now approved by the FDA! There is not one drug that we pushed for earlier access to that did not make it through the clinical trial process. Many lives could have been saved or extended, if there had been earlier access to these drugs!
—Frank Burroughs, Abigail Alliance Founder

If those drugs helped only 10% of the people who took them, 470,000 people might have lived longer lives. If a consumer advocacy group can boast such a good record of predicting which drugs will be effective, one has to wonder why it takes the "experts" at the FDA so long to approve them. The Amendments have made the FDA much more wary of signing off on new drugs because of the scrutiny that the agency will receive if side effects, which every drug has, come to the attention of Congress and the American people.

Exactly how many Americans have died waiting because of the Amendments? We can get an estimate from the number of NCEs approved from 1963 to 1999 and the average increase in development time

Table 1: Lives Lost Because of Amendment-Driven Development Delays

	1963–1969	1970–1979	1980–1989	1990–1999	2000–2009
NCEs approved in each period[5]	83	173	204	290	229
Mean development time in years[6]	8.1	11.6	14.1	14.2	13.1
Extra years caused by the Amendments[7]	4.1	7.6	10.1	10.2	9.1
Millions of life years lost because of Amendment-driven delays[8]	5.0	21.0	36.4	57.8	44.5
Millions of lives lost because of Amendment-driven delays[9]	0.5	1.9	3.3	5.3	4.0
Total Lives Lost (millions)	15.0				

caused by the Amendments (Table 1). After converting life-years saved to lives saved, the total number of lives lost through 2009 resulting from Amendment-driven delays comes to a jaw-dropping 15.0 million. This is 10 times more than the number of Americans who have died in all wars between our country's founding and 2017 (Wikipedia n.d.).

Not all drugs save lives; some simply increase the quality of life by enabling the sick and elderly to live independently or to remain mobile longer. Those who are the least healthy benefit the most from drugs. Because the poor tend to have more illnesses than do the affluent, pharmaceuticals tend to help close the health gap between the rich and the poor (Lichtenberg & Virabhak 2007, 371–92).

No matter how much we practice prevention, eventually our bodies will break down. At that point, drugs may give us a few more years of life. We have not yet learned how to completely foil the Grim Reaper; however, with prevention and treatment together, we are extending our life span. Without the Amendments, our progress would be much faster.

As a research scientist at the Upjohn Co. between 1976 and 1995, I was quite aware of the negative impact of increasing regulatory demands on drug development time. My colleagues and I joked that we spent so much time fulfilling the regulations that we had no time to discover new drugs to treat disease. However, such remarks were "gallows humor" meant to defuse the horror of what was being said. Delays in getting lifesaving drugs to market are no laughing matter. Longer development times are quite literally a matter of life and death.

Most physicians are well aware that too much regulation can be deadly as well. Surveys conducted in the mid-1990s, show that more than two-thirds of neurologists, neurosurgeons, cardiologists, and oncologists agree with this statement: "The FDA is too slow in approving new drugs and medical devices."

When asked if such delays "cost lives by forcing people to go without potentially beneficial therapies," half of the doctors agreed. Depending on the specialty, only 18–36% of physicians felt that the FDA's approval process didn't interfere with their ability to give their patients the best possible care (Competitive Enterprise Institute 1996, 1995).

Clearly, most doctors realize that too much regulation can kill. However, they see the American public as largely unaware of this problem. When asked if the general public understood that "some people may suffer or die waiting for the FDA to act," almost three-quarters of the surveyed physicians disagreed. The remainder felt that the American public had "some" understanding.

You might legitimately ask whether the Amendments saved some lives and wonder how they compare to the deaths caused by Amendment-driven delays. In Chapter 31, we'll compare the lives lost by regulatory delays and loss of innovation to the safety gains from the Amendments. We'll find that death by regulation far exceeds consumer protection, even if the estimates of deaths caused by the Amendments are 100 times too high.

Chapter 11

What Takes So Long?

MANY ARE TRIED, BUT FEW ARE CHOSEN

Someone not involved in drug development might legitimately wonder how it could possibly take so many years to bring a drug to market. When I joined The Upjohn Company in the mid-1970s, I had no idea what was involved. Shortly after I arrived, however, I could hardly believe that any drug actually was able to jump through the maze of ever-changing regulatory hoops and make it to the marketplace.

Company chemists would make 5,000–10,000 potential new drugs, which were then studied in the test tube or other "in vitro" (not in whole animals) to see if they slowed cholesterol synthesis, inhibited a particular enzyme (protein) that helped create disease, or killed the target microbes (PhRMA 2012, 30). Drugs that looked promising might then be tested in animals to see if they worked "in vivo" (in whole animals) with few problematic side effects at the effective doses.

From the original batch of 5,000–10,000 compounds, about 250 began FDA-mandated animal safety testing and other preclinical work. Before passage of the Amendments, pharmaceutical firms—not the FDA—decided which studies were most appropriate.

Somewhere between 3 and 6 years are now consumed by the in vitro, in vivo, and preclinical regulatory and animal safety (toxicology) studies (PhRMA 2012). Because there were only a few instances of too little preclinical testing before passage of the Amendments, it's not clear how much benefit the extended testing provides (Wardell & Lasagna 1975, 20).

The FDA requires specific animal tests before drugs can be tested in people. When I was at Upjohn, the controversial LD50 test had to be performed. Rats and other laboratory animals had to be given enough drug in a single dose to kill half of them. The animals were then examined to discover how the drug killed them. We hoped to find some insight as to what organs were most likely to be affected in people.

After we determined the LD50, a series of sequential animal studies were done at a variety of single and multiple doses to see potential side effects. Those studies took months or years to complete, depending on the drug and the stage of testing.

As the political climate shifted, the actual testing requirements changed during the 14 years or so of development. The regulations became a moving target, making fulfilling them even more difficult.

For example, on one occasion, a scientist from the pathology department recommended that we repeat a whole year of rat toxicology. Toxicology studies test huge doses of drugs in animals in the hopes of discovering which side effects are likely to occur in people. The pathologist told us that the FDA was now "recommending" that all animal toxicology studies use "validated" assays. By the time that we were ready to test our new drug in people, he anticipated that those validated assays would be *required*. If we didn't validate our assays and repeat our animal studies now, they would likely be thrown out a couple of years down the road when we were ready to begin human studies.

An assay measures how much drug is in a particular solution or capsule. Naturally, we already did such tests so we knew how much drug our animals received.

A validated assay was basically the same test. At each step of the process of preparing the drug, however, every instrument had to be meticulously checked for accuracy, and lengthy written logs needed to be kept of the process. We always validated our assays before our drugs were given to people to make sure that they got *exactly* the amount of drug they were supposed to get.

Even without the validation process, our instruments were checked periodically. Consequently, the validated assay usually gave results that were within a couple of percentages of the standard assay.

Validation makes sense before dosing people; you want to be sure that you are giving them exactly the amount of drug intended. From a scientific standpoint, however, validation didn't make much of a difference for toxicology. In those studies, animals routinely got many times what the human dose would be so that side effects could be seen. A difference of a couple of percentages in what the animals received was inconsequential because they were already being greatly overdosed, usually by several hundred percent.

However, the time and expense needed to validate drug assays at the toxicology stage of development was substantial. Only 1 out of every 50 drugs that starts the toxicology process survives the development gauntlet long enough to be tested in humans (PhRMA 2012). By requiring that the validation be done early, its cost was multiplied by a factor of 49 without a compensating gain in safety benefits. In addition, the development process was lengthened by the several weeks or months necessary to set up and complete the meticulous validation process. This is how the development timeline is incrementally increased by the FDA one step at a time.

When a new drug does make it to market, its pricing must include the cost of those 49 validated assays for drugs that never made it into humans or the company would quickly go out of business. By demanding—or even thinking about demanding—tests that don't really increase safety, the FDA needlessly costs consumers a great deal. This waste occurs in many steps along the development pathway, adding greatly to the time and price tag of new drugs.

The FDA became so concerned with checking its regulatory boxes that sometimes they "missed the forest for the trees." When Upjohn became interested in drugs to treat anxiety, we did the normal testing required by the FDA. However, drugs that treat anxiety usually cause some degree of relaxation. At high doses, they induce sleep. Our lab rats slept so long that they starved to death. They simply weren't awake long enough each day to consume what their bodies needed.

This finding should have been good news because the drugs could be taken in high doses without obvious damage to the body, at least in rats. However, the results made the FDA examiners uncomfortable. How could they predict which organs might be affected in people when the drug killed the rats only indirectly by making them sleep too long to eat? How could the next set of animal studies be performed when the dose was supposed to be based on the one that showed side effects? What should have been a cause for celebration became a regulatory concern and held up further progress until this problem had been resolved.

PHASE 3 IS THE MOST-EXPENSIVE HURDLE IN BOTH TIME AND MONEY

Most of the increase in development time and cost came from the growing demands that the FDA made on the number and complexity of human studies. Most new drugs are given to 100 or so healthy volunteers. Blood levels are measured, and side effects are monitored. Those early studies are called Phase 1.

If no major problems are uncovered, more extensive Phase 2 trials might enroll 100 to 500 patients with the targeted disease. Drugs that are well tolerated and show promise of effectiveness then enter into Phase 3 testing. Phase 1–3 was averaging 8.6 years in the 1990s (DiMasi 2001a).

Because the Amendments directed the FDA to allow only effective drugs on the market, the FDA had to define what "effective" meant. The FDA chose a high standard of proof: a drug had to show that it was better than a placebo in two separate human Phase 3 studies. Until recently, the FDA would accept studies done only in the United States. "Better than placebo" was defined as "statistically significant at the $p<0.05$ level."

To understand what that definition means, consider a drug that lowers blood pressure. If 10 people are treated with it and if *every* person experienced a blood pressure drop of 5 mm, we would be almost certain that the drug lowered blood pressure. When we did the math, the statistics would show "almost certain" as a "p" value of 0.05 or less ($p<0.05$). This finding means that there is a 95% chance that the drug really works and a 5% chance that what we saw was a chance occurrence.

As you might expect, real life isn't so systematic. We are all different in a number of ways: different genetics, different fitness levels, different diets, and different ages. Consequently, a drug that lowers blood pressure doesn't work the same way in everyone; only about 30–50% of patients see favorable results (Norton 2001, 180–85; Conner 2011).

Blood pressure is controlled by the body in several ways; anti-hypertensive drugs work on the various points of control. A person's high blood pressure can be caused by a problem in one place or in several. Usually, we don't know where the problem is. Some people will respond to the medication and others won't, but we usually can't predict to which group a particular individual will belong.

Consequently, in real life when we test a blood pressure medicine, some people get no benefit at all. Others might experience a 10 mm drop in blood pressure; some 5 mm; some only 3mm. A few might find that their blood pressure actually goes up 3 mm because of their unique body biochemistry. In the placebo group, some people will also experience a drop or increase in blood pressure because of the placebo effect.

With all that variation, how can we tell if the two groups are really different? We use statistics to find out. Statistics is a mathematical way of estimating the probability that the placebo and treated groups are different. If the statistics tell us that we are 95% confident that the drug really works, we say that the drug is effective.

Why 95%? Why not 90% or even 80%? Basically, the answer is scientific tradition. It's quite arbitrary. It's also such a high standard that the number of people in the drug group and the placebo group must be quite large to see effectiveness at the $p<0.05$ level. Most clinical studies designed to show effectiveness involve hundreds of people and take several years to perform.

Statistics show the 95% certainty best when every person has the same drop in blood pressure, even if it's small. If the drug works on only one point of control, it might cause a large drop in three people, but not affect the other seven at all. Some people might benefit greatly by such a drug, but statistics might not show a 95% certainty. If so, a drug that could save lives could easily be discarded as ineffective.

A drug that lowers blood pressure a small amount in everyone might be "statistically significant" but might not have any real positive effect on a person's health. We call that "clinically insignificant." Conversely, a drug that lowered blood pressure greatly in a small number of people might have a remarkable positive effect on their health, but it won't always show a "statistically significant" outcome because only a small percentage of people will be helped.

The number of people in a study makes a big difference in statistical outcome too. Because drug companies can only guess at how many people they might need to get statistical significance, they must often repeat time-consuming and expensive studies when they guess wrong. Critics of the pharmaceutical companies complain that many clinical trials fail to show a drug works and that drug companies report only positive results. Many times the negative results are simply the failure of earlier trials to attain statistical significance. In other words, the drug works, but too few people were enrolled in earlier trials to achieve the $p<0.05$ level that is the traditional cutoff for effectiveness.

Phase 3 studies typically involve thousands of diseased patients from several places around the country or even around the world. The FDA usually requires statistically significant effectiveness from not one but two Phase 3 trials. For researchers to increase the chances of getting statistically significant results, the patients in the studies are matched as carefully as possible so that they are similar in terms of age, medical condition, sex, and other factors that could influence the outcome.

The complexity of the trials increases every year as the FDA demands more and more data for each study. The work burden per study grew 65–80% in the first decade of the 21st century (Allison 2012, 41–49; Getz & Kaitin 2015, 3–15), almost doubling the cost of human testing (DiMasi, Grabowski, & Hansen 2016).

In recent years, the FDA has also insisted on "outcome studies" lasting 2–3 years. Even if a drug lowers blood sugar, for example, the FDA will not always assume that it helps diabetics. The manufacturer (drug company) must demonstrate that it significantly reduces heart attacks, strokes, or other problems that diabetics have.

As a result, the average human testing time for diabetic drugs approved in the United States has risen two full years since the year 2000 (DiMasi 2015). From 2005 to 2010, the number of patients in those trials more than doubled (Viereck & Boudes 2011, 324–32).

For anti-obesity drugs, the FDA wants long-term studies that look at cardiovascular events (LaMattina 2013, 34–37). For anti-inflammatory drugs, the FDA wants to see 1–3 year studies measuring overall health outcomes (LaMattina 2013, 110–11). Naturally, all of those regulatory demands increase the development time and cost of taking a new drug to market. Higher costs mean higher pharmacy prices, as we'll see in Chapter 18.

The FDA has tightened up the requirements for approving new drugs for adult-onset diabetes, a disease that affects approximately 25 million Americans. The result is that performing the clinical trials for a new diabetes drug is so long and costly that no venture capital firm will finance a new diabetes drug … no venture capital firm will finance a new effort to develop a drug for the obesity epidemic.

—Dr. John Freund, Skyline Ventures, a capital firm specializing in biopharmaceutical drug companies

DRUGS AREN'T HOME FREE EVEN AFTER PHASE 3

Even after completion of successful Phase 3 trials, a drug still has to jump some regulatory hurdles. First, the FDA must review the truckload of studies compiled by the drug company, which today are sent electronically. The FDA's review process usually takes more than a year (Kaitlin & Cairns 2003, 357–71). Only one out of every six drugs that enter clinical testing will actually be approved for marketing (PhRMA 2012, 30).

Once the drug is approved—or before that if the drug company feels confident—manufacturing facilities must be put in place. Even if an old line will be converted to accommodate the newly approved pharmaceutical, tweaks must be made, and an elaborate validation and recordkeeping process—known as GMP, or Good Manufacturing Practices—must be put in place. The FDA can inspect the new line and insist on changes.

In addition, the company must negotiate the labeling for the new drug. The FDA reviews the wording that goes on the box or label, the package insert that goes into the box, the wording of ads, the information that pharmaceutical representatives can and cannot share with the doctors they visit, and every piece of advertising copy. The FDA does not believe that "commercial speech" is protected by the First Amendment of the US Constitution; instead, the agency claims jurisdiction over what information drug companies are allowed to share. The process of approving the advertising and labeling can take many months of back and forth between the FDA and the drug company.

Finally, the FDA generally requires follow-up studies after the drug is marketed, especially if it is concerned that side effects that didn't show up in the limited human testing will become visible when large numbers of people take the drug. Those postmarketing studies are known as Phase 4. As mentioned earlier, Britain has historically put more emphasis on Phase 4 than on the animal work and lengthy premarket human studies that the FDA favors.

Chapter 12

The Amendments Put Small Firms Out of Business

The increased cost of getting new drugs to market means that a company can lose hundreds of millions, if not billions, of dollars (Chapter 17) if a new drug isn't approved or drops out in late stage development. Clearly, only a large company can handle this kind of loss without having to declare bankruptcy. Pharmaceutical companies have had to merge to survive the increasing post-Amendment development regulatory costs.

Although the "merger mania" of today is creating a pharmaceutical cartel of a few big players, the Amendments have been putting small firms out of business ever since they were passed. The smaller companies, which were the most-efficient producers of new drugs before 1962, were the first to go.

Before 1963, the smallest firms (fewer than 1,000 employees) required only 80% of the resources of large firms (5,000+ employees) to produce the same amount of R&D (Jadlow 1970, 160–61). Large firms took about three times as long to develop drugs compared to those produced by smaller companies and had costs about eight times as high (Jadlow 1970, 38).

Drawing on my experience, I suspect smaller firms were more efficient because of their more streamlined management. Although the

Upjohn Company was considered to be a medium-sized firm during my years there, I always felt that the many layers of management led to considerable inefficiency.

As early as 1966, Amendment-related costs for the large firms had increased about 24%, but the small firms were spending 70% more to produce the same amount of R&D as they had pre-Amendment (Jadlow 1970, 160). The larger firms enjoyed more economies of scale than the small ones did, even though their costs increased too.

Clearly, small firms were at a disadvantage after the passage of the Amendments. Many went out of businesses. Between 1955 and 1962, the smallest 98% of US drug firms brought 12% of the industry's self-originated drugs to market; between 1963 and 1966, they produced no new drugs (Jadlow 1970, 175–88). By 1968, the number of firms introducing new drugs into the marketplace had plummeted by 44% (Jadlow 1970, 176; Sarett 1974). The cartelization of the pharmaceutical industry had begun. As the smaller firms vanished, the larger firms became the sole source of NCEs. In 1962, 108 firms introduced new pharmaceuticals. By 1968, only 48 firms did so (Mund 1970, 125–38).

The Amendments gave the FDA more authority over the manufacturing process as well as development. The FDA performed site inspections and demanded to see documents that some companies objected to, especially after one FDA employee was indicted for sharing one company's trade secrets with another (Jondrow 1972, 89). The regulators' access to company trade secrets created opportunities for corruption.

In 1963, the FDA established the Good Manufacturing Practices (GMP) Regulations, which were designed to document each step of a drug's manufacturing process, starting from the purchase of the raw materials from which it was made. Along the way, checks were made for purity and the amount of drug in each dosing unit. The instruments used for those measurements also had to undergo extensive documented testing to ensure their accuracy. Many checks were redundant. The person who did them had to sign the documentation. The FDA could specify exactly which records had to be kept, and it could withdraw drug approvals if manufacturers failed to comply (Jondrow 1972, 15–16).

It was no longer sufficient to show that the final product matched what was stated on the bottle. If, along the way, the newly mandated documentation was not in place, the FDA could claim that defective batches were likely and could stop them from being marketed (Jondrow 1972, 27–28). Through the GMP process, the FDA began dictating the educational level and experience of manufacturing personnel as well (Jondrow 1972, 29).

Moreover, the FDA lowered the allowable variation in penicillin potency below that which manufacturers had been using. The FDA even proposed that each machine on the manufacturing line be dedicated to a single drug (Jondrow 1972, 88–89). Clearly, such changes, when implemented, hurt the small manufacturers more than the large ones.

In 1968, the FDA began its intensified inspections of companies that had the poorest recall records. Such inspections often took several months. The FDA completed 191 inspections between 1968 and 1970. Moreover, 23% of companies failed to meet the FDA's standards. Half of those were forced out of business immediately, while the other half sued (Jondrow 1972, 72–73). As the smaller drug companies went out of business, the lack of competition—along with the additional costs posed by the Amendments—allowed larger firms to raise prices on their new NCEs.

In Britain, where regulations hadn't increased as much, small firms continued to thrive; however, price increases on new drugs were much lower than in the United States (LG Thomas 1990). By creating a pharmaceutical cartel, the Amendments thus increased costs to the consumer.

The absorption of smaller companies into the larger ones created cuts in R&D as redundant workers were let go. Productivity declined as workers became discouraged with the possibility of being downsized (LaMattina 2013, 32–34). In 1988, the Pharmaceutical Research and Manufacturing Association (PhRMA, formerly the PMA) still boasted

42 companies. By 2012, most of those companies had been bought out or merged: only 11 of the original 42 remained (LaMattina 2013, 27–29).

If this trend continues—and it will unless we fix the problems behind the Amendments—a handful of very large corporations will choose which drugs will undergo development. Although some small biotechnology firms still attempt to take drugs all the way from discovery to FDA approval, most still depend on the bigger companies to assume the heavy lifting during the later stages of the development process. Today, much of the innovation comes from those smaller companies, which take most of the research risk.

Industry consolidation of the last 15 years has resulted in less competition, less investment in R&D, and a gradual decrease in the approval of new medicines.
—John L. LaMattina, former president of Pfizer's Global R&D

In 2000, the FDA intensified its GMP demands, specifically on vaccine manufacturers, who claimed they were not given adequate notice of the new requirements. Companies had to upgrade their equipment, even if was working perfectly, and they were fined for any violations in record-keeping. The FDA didn't find any contaminated vaccines or product problems during those inspections, but its increasing demands made vaccines unprofitable for some manufacturers, who naturally stopped making them. When vaccine shortages cropped up as a result, the FDA remarked that the firms had stopped producing vaccines as a result of business decisions. However, the agency temporarily backed off its GMP enforcement, possibly because of such unanticipated consequences, without actually changing any of the rules it had already made (Foulkes 2004, 31–54).

Wall Street analysts, more interested in short-term outcomes than long-term ones, are encouraging the industry to cut back even further on R&D. They actually criticized Merck when its CEO, Kenneth Frazier, wanted to increase investment in innovation. "Merck could end up wasting billions of dollars" was typical of the critique that sent Merck's stock downward (LaMattina 2011).

Pfizer pleased Wall Street by decreasing its R&D to a mere 11% of its sales dollar in 2012 (LaMattina 2013, 29), which is about half of the industry average (PhRMA 2013, ii). Pfizer's stock price rose as a result (LaMattina 2013, 112). Less R&D means less innovation, fewer new drugs, and more premature deaths.

Chapter 13

Rules Are for Thee, But Not for Me

On almost any aspect of drug regulation that one chooses to examine, there is usually an extraordinarily wide variation in philosophy and operational procedures from division to division and even from reviewer to reviewer.
—Louis Lasagna, Tufts University

Chapter 11 may give the impression that the FDA seeks to apply a rigorous and consistent standard to the drugs it approves. However, FDA decisions are ultimately based on political nuances as much as—or more than—on the science. Some drugs are rushed through the process because their champions are other government agencies or drug companies with which the FDA enjoys a good rapport. Small biotechnology firms can be bankrupted when the FDA requires more studies than they have anticipated. The history of drugs intended to treat AIDS patients provides a good illustration of the variability in requirements for drug approval.

AZT

When the AIDS epidemic began, the US pharmacist had little to offer its unfortunate victims. Consequently, AIDS patients began bringing in antiviral drugs or immune stimulants that were approved in other nations, such as ribavirin and isoprinosine. It might have made sense to approve those drugs on the basis of data from other countries, but back then the FDA insisted on considering only studies done in the United States. Today, the agency will consider data from other nations.

Azidothymidine (AZT) had been synthesized in 1964 and tested for anti-cancer activity primarily through funding from the National Cancer Institute (NCI) (Horwitz, Chua, & Noe 1964, 2076–79), a division of the National Institutes of Health (NIH). The NIH is the primary government agency that distributes grants to universities, hospitals, and other research institutions for biomedical research. When AZT failed as an anti-cancer agent, it was set aside.

Ten years later, Wofram Ostertag at the Max Planck Institute in Germany showed that AZT could inhibit the growth of the Friend leukemia retrovirus in cell culture (Ostertag, Roesler, Krieg, et al. 1974, 4980–85). In 1983, scientists at the Pasteur Institute in Paris and the NCI in the United States proposed that the human immunodeficiency virus (HIV), also a retrovirus, was the cause of AIDS (Barré-Sinoussi, Chermann, Rey, et al. 1983, 868–71; Popovic, Sarngadharan, Read, et al. 1984, 497–500; Gallo, Salahuddin, Popovic, et al. 1984, 500–03; Schüpbach, Popovic, Gilden, et al. 1984, 503–05; Sarngadharan, Popovic, Bruch, et al. 1984, 506–08).

Shortly thereafter, NCI scientists developed an assay to screen for drugs that protected $CD4^+$ T cells, an important component of the immune system, from attack by the HIV virus (Mitsuya, Popovic, Yarchoan, et al. 1984, 172–74). NCI asked companies to submit their most-promising anti-viral compounds for testing and to commit to developing those drugs if they were active against HIV.

Pharmaceutical firms kept vast libraries of all kinds of drugs, including anti-viral compounds, but they had not yet invested in the expensive containment facilities necessary to handle the HIV virus without endangering their researchers. At this beginning stage in the AIDS epidemic, many companies felt that the small number of patients identified with the disease might make recovering the high post-Amendment development costs prohibitive.

One pharmaceutical firm, Burroughs-Wellcome, used the less-dangerous Friend and Harvey sarcoma retroviruses to test for potential activity against HIV. They were especially interested in drugs such as AZT that would inhibit reverse transcriptase, an enzyme required for the retroviruses to reproduce. Along with 10 other drugs, Burroughs-Wellcome sent AZT to the NCI for testing against the HIV virus. Burroughs-Wellcome would later use this selection process to make a patent claim for AZT's utility in AIDS.

In February 1985, NCI scientists found that the AZT sent to them by Burroughs-Wellcome inhibited the growth of HIV in the test tube (Mitsuya, Weinhold, Furman, et al. 1985, 7096–100). Several months later, NCI organized a Phase 1 trial of AZT at Duke University. AZT increased the CD4$^+$ T cells in AIDS patients, who improved enough to regain some of their lost weight (Yarchoan, Klecker, Weinhold, et al. 1986, 575–80).

After such encouraging results, Burroughs-Wellcome took over the more intensive phases of AZT development. The company initiated a double-blind, placebo-controlled Phase 2 trial of AZT involving 282 AIDS patients (Fischl, Richman, Grieco, et al. 1987, 185–91). Although neither the doctors nor the patients were told who got active drug and who got placebo, patients were able to tell by the way they felt who was getting AZT (Kwitny 1992, 167). Although 19 placebo patients died during the study, only 1 who received AZT did (p<0.001). Once AZT was found to be more effective than placebo, even in this single study, giving placebo to AIDS patients became ethically questionable.

Penicillin couldn't get through that fast.
—James Todd, senior vice president of the American Medical Association, referring to AZT

In an unprecedented move, the FDA waived Phase 3 trials and approved AZT on March 20, 1987, just 25 months after the first demonstration that AZT was active against HIV in the test tube (Cimons 1987). Such short development times from laboratory bench to market were common before the Amendments, but unheard of after their passage.

AZT's approval made an end run around the post-Amendment criteria, presumably because another federal agency was so heavily involved. Other drugs, such as isoprinosine and ribavirin (see later), marketed extensively elsewhere, did not get the preferential treatment accorded AZT. Because those drugs delayed the development of full-blown AIDS in HIV-positive patients, they actually prevented the need for more intensive treatment. Also, they usually exhibited fewer side effects than AZT did.

We have been denied access to drugs that have passed Phase 2 placebo-controlled trials to the satisfaction of [government-approved] investigators, drugs that have been proven to the satisfaction of independent world-class experts. We have experienced a system that has delivered a single drug [AZT], which has proven both far more toxic and far less effective than they told us.
—Martin Delaney, California AIDS activist responsible for
one of the largest buyers clubs

ISOPRINOSINE

Isoprinosine was one of the drugs that AIDS patients brought into the United States from other countries. In the 1970s, Newport Pharmaceuticals' founder, Dr. Alvin J. Glasky, discovered isoprinosine and documented its immune-boosting qualities against a form of encephalitis. Glasky asked the FDA for permission to distribute the drug free of charge to victims, but the FDA refused to permit this practice because isoprinosine hadn't been put through its approval process. Appalled, Glasky tried to sue the FDA. The courts, of course, told Glasky that the FDA had carte blanche (Kwitny 1992, 101).

In December 1985, *The Lancet* published a paper written by several doctors, including NCI's Robert C. Gallo, who had helped to link the HIV virus to AIDS. They found that isoprinosine prevented the virus from infecting and killing T-cells in a test tube (Pompidou, Zagury, Gallo, et al. 1985, 1423). If the drug worked the same way in people, it might protect patients infected with HIV from ever developing the full-blown disease.

New Zealand immediately approved isoprinosine to treat HIV-positive patients. Because the FDA didn't, the US AIDS community continued buying the drug in Mexico (Kwitny 1992, 102). The drug was marketed in more than 80 countries for other indications and had a good safety record (Hanley 1986).

Glasky went back to the FDA, which approved a study on patients who had the HIV virus that hadn't yet progressed to full-blown AIDS. CD4+T-cell counts were used to measure isoprinosine's effectiveness.

T-cells circulate in the blood and are an important part of our immune system. In AIDS patients, CD4+T cell numbers went down, but no one knew (yet) if they could truly predict the course of the disease. Usually, the FDA did not like using those "surrogate markers" as a basis for approving a drug. Surrogate markers don't measure the endpoint (death) that the FDA hopes the drug addresses, but they measure something that is assumed to predict it. Of course, this particular surrogate marker was the same one used in the AZT human studies, which resulted in the drug's rapid approval.

Even though isoprinosine protected the CD4+T-cell count from deteriorating, the FDA claimed that Newport's study was irrelevant. The FDA wanted to see studies showing that the virus had been killed throughout the body or that the treated patients lived longer than untreated ones, even though the agency hadn't held AZT to that standard. In frustration, Glasky denounced the FDA in a press conference, essentially killing isoprinosine's chances for approval in the foreseeable future (Kwitny 1992, 102–03).

… isoprinsoine is one of the drugs of choice for AIDS. It's a crime that politics is going to keep it from ever being used in the U.S. In order to get a drug approved, you have to have the NIH Mafia behind it.
—Dr. Alvin J. Glasky, Newport Pharmaceuticals

About 4 years later, a Scandinavian research group published its findings. After 24 weeks, 17 of the 403 placebo patients progressed from HIV infection to AIDS. Only 2 of the 412 isoprinosine-treated patients did. No serious side effects were observed (Pedersen, Sandstrom, Petersen, et al. 1990, 1757–63). Had the FDA approved isoprinosine on the basis of T-cell counts, thousands of HIV patients might never have developed AIDS. Isoprinsoine has fewer side effects than AZT does, which makes it more appropriate for long-term preventative treatment (Kwitny 1992, 146).

Let's pretend that we had decided in 1986 to accept surrogate markers. Now, look back at every drug in every study we've had since then and ask yourself these questions: is there any drug we would have approved inappropriately based on the markers? Or is there any drug we would've rejected inappropriately? Would we have made any mistakes? If the answer to that is no—as we believe it is—then we have wasted 6 years.
—Martin Delaney, prominent AIDS activist speaking at a
FDA Advisory Committee meeting in 1991

RIBAVIRIN

Ribavirin is an anti-viral drug sold in many countries worldwide. The AIDs community began smuggling this drug in from Mexico, because it wasn't marketed in the United States. Publications documenting its safety profile and its activity against a number of viruses had been appearing in the scientific literature since the early 1970s (Kwitny 1992, 78).

An aerosolized version of the drug was approved in December 31, 1985, for treatment of infants with respiratory syncytial virus (RSV) (US FDA Annual Ed.). Ribavirin's manufacturer, ICN Pharmaceuticals, got on the wrong side of the FDA when announcing its approval by truthfully indicating that the drug was marketed worldwide for a number of infections (Lindren 1986). The FDA considered such statements to be misleading advertising, because the ribavirin had not gotten FDA approval for use against anything but RSV.

In January 1987, ICN announced the results of "the longest and most-extensive trials ever held to test the potential anti-viral activity of any drug against the AIDS virus." After 24 weeks of treatment, none of the 52 HIV-positive patients treated with 800 mg of ribavirin had gone on to develop full-blown AIDS. Of the 55 patients who were dosed with 600 mg of the drug, 6 developed AIDS, as did 10 of the 56 placebo-treated patients (Altman 1987).

Shortly after ICN's press conference, criticism of the FDA's study began to appear in the press (Kwitny 1992, 147). FDA Commissioner Frank Young stopped further ribavirin studies because of "safety concerns" and "insufficient evidence of effectiveness," which basically halted ribavirin's US development program (Kwitny 1992, 155). Dr. Ellen Cooper, who did most of the reviews for the AIDS drugs, implied that the sickest patients in the ICN study had been put into the placebo group. She told Congress that the drug might actually accelerate the development of AIDS (Kwitny 1992, 155–57). On the basis of those claims, ICN was accused of securities fraud (Crouch 1991), which could have resulted in prison time for some of ICN's management.

In June 1987 at the Third International Conference on AIDS, Dr. Peter Mansell presented the actual data from the study, which indicated that the drug worked. During the question and answer session, FDA Commissioner Frank Young came up to the podium, introduced himself, and claimed that he had seen no evidence of ribavirin's effectiveness (Kwitny 1992, 158–60). Shortly afterward, he sent an investigator to determine whether ethics violations had occurred during the study (Kwitny 1992, 183).

Later, a packet of papers surfaced, indicating that the FDA had known of several independent evaluations of the study's data, including that of David Cox, who had developed the statistical Cox test used to interpret it. All agreed that ICN had treated the data appropriately, while the FDA's interpretation was "almost ludicrous" and "possibly disingenuous" (Kwitny 1992, 181–84). This information, showing that the FDA attacks had been groundless, was passed on to then–Vice

President Bush. Four days later, presumably caused by political pressure exerted by Bush, the FDA quietly allowed ICN to resume human testing (Kwitny 1992, 187).

In the summer of 1990, the ribavirin study, which the FDA had maligned, was published in a prestigious peer-reviewed journal and addressed the FDA's criticisms (Roberts, Dickinson, Heseltine, et al. 1990, 884–92). However, by that time, ICN had given up trying to get the drug approved for AIDS in the United States (Berkman 1990).

Who could blame ICN? For trying to make a drug to stop the development of AIDS, members of its management were rewarded with criminal charges, accusations of unethical conduct, and distortion of their data analysis. Poisonous politics had infected the drug approval process, thus discouraging innovators who might otherwise have been able to offer the AIDS community some hope.

There was talk that no treatment or vaccine would get quick FDA approval for experimentation unless it was developed by the federal government; among AIDS organizers, NIH had become the acronym for the agency disinterested in treatments that were Not Invented Here. There was no stop the government did not pull out for AZT, the drug the NCI had originally developed. However, there seemed to be no bit of red tape too minor to delay the release of other treatments.
—Randy Shilts in his book, *And the Band Played On: Politics, People, and the AIDS Epidemic,* 2007

GANCICLOVIR

About half of the US population harbors the CMV (cytomegalovirus retinitis) virus, which is usually suppressed by our body's own defenses. However, in AIDS patients and others with a compromised immune system, it rages unchecked, causing inflammation of the retina and, eventually, blindness.

In 1980, Syntex synthesized a drug that became known as ganciclovir, which specifically targeted CMV. Syntax got permission from the FDA in 1984 to give away the drug to doctors who requested it while development was ongoing. Burroughs-Wellcome had its own version of the drug. Together, the two companies distributed enough anti-CMV drugs to treat 6,300 people. As hoped, the drug prevented many of the AIDS victims from going blind.

In 1987, Syntex submitted the anecdotal data to the FDA, asking for approval. No double-blind, placebo-controlled studies had been conducted. Indeed, such studies would likely have been considered unethical, because they would have deprived the placebo-treated group from a treatment that everyone now knew worked. Nevertheless, the advisory committee reluctantly voted not to approve ganciclovir without the required studies.

The FDA tried to design a protocol with placebo controls that would pass muster with the ethicists, but it was unable to do so. In an attempt to force the issue, the FDA threatened to stop Syntex from giving the drug away. Had the FDA succeeded in either of those endeavors, hundreds—perhaps thousands—of AIDS patients would have had to go blind in order for the regulatory boxes to be checked.

The outcry from the AIDS community convinced the FDA to allow Syntex to keep up its free distribution of ganciclovir. Finally, the FDA approved the drug in 1989 with basically the same data that Syntex submitted in 1987 and without a double-blind, placebo-controlled study (Burkholz 1994, 117–22). Clearly, the FDA is influenced, for better or worse, by political pressures and publicity.

PENTAMIDINE

In the 1980s, almost 80% of US AIDS patients came down with a deadly form of pneumonia known as PCP (Pneumocystis pneumonia).

The disease caused scarring of the lungs, so victims could survive only two or three attacks before dying. The intravenous drug, pentamidine, used primarily to prevent African sleeping sickness, was able to treat PCP, which had been a rare disease before hitting the AIDS community.

Supplies of the drug were limited to a sole British manufacturer, because the demand had been small. The Centers for Disease Control and Prevention (CDC) in Atlanta made its limited supplies available in the United States as needed, but the AIDS epidemic created too large a demand for the CDC to service. The CDC had difficulty convincing a US drug company to manufacture it. The Amendments had made patents necessary to recover development costs, and pentamidine's patent had expired.

Finally, a Chicago-based drug company, Lyphomed, was induced to produce supplies for PCP under the Orphan Drug Act. The development costs created by the Amendments were so high that drugs for diseases with small populations had no chance of recovering their costs and were therefore orphaned. The act allowed the FDA to lower the standards for effectiveness and to grant the developer a 7-year monopoly after an orphan drug's approval. Even if another company developed a drug for the same orphaned population, that company couldn't market its drug unless it was better than the drug given orphan status (Public Law 97-414).

Because the effectiveness of pentamidine in PCP had already been established, the FDA waived the usual clinical trials for Lyphomed. In the fall of 1984, intravenous pentamidine gained FDA approval.

However, at least in AIDS patients, the intravenous route usually didn't get enough of the drug to the lungs before toxic reactions were observed. Animal studies showed that aerosolized pentamidine put the drug right where it was needed—in the lungs—and was safer.

The FDA considered aerosolized pentamidine, which was a new drug and was required to go through the normal development process. The NIH tried to organize some of the required trials, but it didn't actually enroll patients until March 1988. Although the NIH could organize a small Phase 1 study, a Phase 2 or Phase 3 trial was more challenging. Patients didn't want to enroll in a study where they had only a 50:50 chance of receiving placebo instead of the drug that was likely to save their sight.

Instead, the underground AIDS community put together supplies of the aerosolized drug and illegally circulated them for prevention of PCP. In the summer of 1989, the FDA approved aerosolized pentamidine, in part on the basis of its positive experience in the AIDS community (Burkholz 1994, 113–17).

BLOOD TESTS FOR HIV

When NCI's Dr. Robert Gallo developed a blood test for HIV, the FDA took just a few months to approve it. However, Gallo considered even that short delay to be deadly. He argued that the test should be used to screen the US blood supply. Even an imperfect test, he claimed, would be better than none at all.

The FDA disagreed and wouldn't permit the test to be used. Meanwhile, Japan continued to import US blood supplies for hemophiliacs. In the 3 months following the FDA's refusal to allow testing of blood supplies, the HIV infection rate in Japan rose from 0% to 13% (Kwitny 1992, 349–50). What happens in the United States ripples outward into the rest of the world, causing harm overseas as well as at home.

The FDA's 3-month delay in approving Gallo's blood test for screening of the US blood supply caused considerable tragedy. However, the agency's 5-year delay in approving essentially the same test packaged for home use by a Johnson & Johnson subsidiary was even more lethal. The HIV home test kit cost under $40, making it affordable for just about anyone who suspected he or she might have been infected. At the time, testing in a doctor's office or clinic cost hundreds of dollars. One researcher estimated that about 10,000 Americans, or 10% of the US AIDS population, were needlessly infected during the delay because their partners were unaware that they were carriers (Goldberg 1997).

As with AZT, the FDA moved the product of another government agency rapidly through its regulatory red tape, while needlessly stalling for years when a similar test was developed by a private firm. Needless to say, such favoritism had many companies reconsidering their commitment to AIDS research.

Chapter 14

Congress Acknowledges Regulations Account for Half of Drug Development Time

A s drug development times increased, so did the costs (Chapter 17). Without a patent, which allowed a company several years of monopoly, it would be difficult—if not impossible—to recover the costs. Shortly after I began my pharmaceutical career in the mid-1970s, Upjohn management directed researchers not to propose any drugs for development that were not patentable. Other companies made the same decision so they could stay solvent.

Although patents had been a prominent feature of the drug industry for decades before the Amendments, products without patents could sometimes be profitable. However, as costs of development rose as a result of the Amendments, patents went from an option to a necessity.

Patents took several years to obtain; companies applied for patents to cover entire families of compounds even before they knew which of the unique chemical structures might be selected for development. In most cases, the patents would be granted before the drugs were marketed. Patents generally expired 17 years from the grant date, not from the date of FDA approval, so the effective patent length when marketing began was considerably less than 17 years. When the patent expired, generic manufacturers could step in.

As development times increased, the effective patent life of an NCE went from 11.4 years in 1976 to a mere 6.8 years in 1981 (Wardell 1983). Consequently, manufacturers had to charge higher prices for new drugs within this shorter window of time to recover their ever-increasing R&D costs.

To counter this trend, Congress passed the Waxman Hatch Patent Restoration Act in 1984 to extend pharmaceutical patent life (Shulman, DiMasi, & Kaitin 1999, 63–68). As we'll see in Chapter 24, the number of new drugs granted FDA approval had fallen off precipitously after the passage of the Amendments. Congress thought that giving drug companies more time to recoup their development costs might encourage more drug innovation.

The Waxman Hatch Act allowed companies to recover some of the "regulatory review time" up to a period of 5 years, as long as the total patent life at the time of marketing didn't exceed 14 years. The Act defined the regulatory review time as the time taken by the FDA's review of the data plus one-half of the years of clinical testing. For the 1980s, the regulatory review time was 7.3 years or 52% of the 14.1 years of development time (DiMasi 2001a, 292, Figure 5).

The regulatory review time, as defined by the Waxman-Hatch Act, greatly underestimated the amount of development time needed to satisfy the regulations, because it didn't count the extra studies demanded by the FDA prior to clinical testing and counted only one-half of the extensive clinical trials that were required after 1962. As Figure 1 illustrates, the Amendments more than tripled development time, so about 70% of the total development time around the turn of the century was due solely to the Amendments.

The Waxman-Hatch regulatory review time was adjusted downward if the manufacturer let the development program languish between the start of testing and issuance of the patent. After all of the nuances were taken into consideration, the average new drug approved from 1993 to 1995 gained 3 years of patent life (Shulman, DiMasi, & Kaitin 1999). As a trade-off to the generic companies that were hurt by this new legislation, the Waxman-Hatch Act also made it easier for generic drugs to enter the market when the patents expired.

Chapter 15

Lifesaving Information for Older Drugs Is Delayed

Sometimes, we don't realize how lifesaving a drug can be until long after it's been marketed. The Amendments created delays in getting information to both doctors and patients about new, lifesaving uses of older, off-patent drugs.

For example, in 1969, the Squibb Chemical Company wanted to study and promote aspirin for prevention of heart disease and stroke. When the FDA told the firm what it had to do under the Amendments, Squibb became discouraged. Because aspirin was off-patent, the company knew that it probably couldn't recover the additional development costs required, and it chose not to perform the necessary studies (Ricardo-Campbell 1976, 48). Without those studies, manufacturers could not legally tell the American public about aspirin's lifesaving effects, because the FDA would consider such information unapproved labeling and prosecute them.

A pharmaceutical firm might have FDA approval to sell a drug for treating one disease, but the FDA still forbids the company from talking to doctors or the public about new, innovative uses for this drug without additional expensive and time-consuming studies. As a result, the company is often better off financially to start over with a brand new drug that has patent protection so it has a chance to recover the extra costs.

Because of the FDA's Amendment-driven restrictions, most Americans were unaware in the late 1960s that they might be able to prevent heart attacks and stroke by taking a low dose of daily aspirin. Not many physicians were aware of aspirin's benefits either.

However, The Upjohn Company, a few other pharmaceutical firms, and several university laboratories were studying aspirin's positive and negative effects on prostaglandins, which are now more commonly referred to as eicosanoinds. Those short-lived hormones are made in virtually every cell in the body. They operate in a yin–yang fashion: some increase blood pressure, for example, and some lower it. Some, such as thromboxane (TxB_2), make the clotting component of blood (platelets) form clumps; some, such as prostacyclin (PGI_2), keep them from doing so. Too much TxB_2 creates clots that stop the flow of blood in the arteries or veins in which they occur. Too much PGI_2 causes uncontrolled bleeding. Our bodies maintain balance by the proper mix of the opposing eicosanoids. Anti-inflammatory drugs, such as aspirin and ibuprofen, alter this balance.

One day, Dr. James W. Aiken, an Upjohn colleague, asked me to come up to his laboratory to see a remarkable experiment. An anesthetized dog lay open on his surgical table with a tie around a coronary artery leading to its heart. By tightening the string, my colleague mimicked the narrowing of the coronary artery that occurs when cholesterol plaque builds up inside of it. Platelets flowing through a narrowed coronary artery are more likely to clump. The clot dramatically slows or even stops blood flow to the heart, causing what we refer to as a heart attack.

By tightening the string around the coronary artery and causing the platelets to clot, my colleague was able to induce heart attacks in sleeping dogs. When he infused PGI_2 into a dog's blood stream, however, the platelets wouldn't clump. In dogs that didn't get PGI_2, the clots that formed could be *dissolved* simply by dripping some PGI_2 on the blocked artery (Aiken, Gorman, & Shebuski 1979, 483–94).

Those experiments suggested that if we could give a drug that increased PGI_2, that decreased TxB_2, or both, we could decrease the chance of a heart attack or even stop one in progress. Fortunately, such a drug was readily available.

Aspirin, the humble over-the-counter drug found in virtually every American household, prevents heart attacks by tweaking the eicosanoid balance to produce more PGI_2 and less TxB_2. Taking an aspirin during a heart attack may stop it from getting worse or may even help resolve it. Consequently, aspirin has become an essential part of a cardiologist's medicine chest (Vandvik, Gutterman, Alonso-Coello, et al. 2012, e637S–e668S).

Sadly, Americans died needlessly from heart problems for 20 years because they were unaware that heart attacks and stroke could be prevented by routine consumption of aspirin. Then, 20 years after the FDA's regulatory requirements discouraged Squibb from studying and promoting aspirin's benefits, US taxpayers—via the National Institutes of Health—funded a landmark study on aspirin (Steering Committee of the Physicians' Health Study Research Group 1989, 129–35).

Published in 1989, this study followed 22,000 male physicians who took aspirin every other day. Heart attacks were reduced by a whopping 44% in doctors older than 50 (Steering Committee 1989). The study was supposed to continue for 10 years but was stopped after 5 because of the dramatic results. The investigators felt it would be unethical to continue to give placebo when aspirin could clearly prevent heart attacks. The results and subsequent confirming studies (Vandvik, Gutterman, Alonso-Coello, et al. 2012; Berger, Roncaglioni, Avanzini, et al. 2006, 306–13) spurred a 500% increase in aspirin use by the mid-1990s (Heidenreich & McClellan 2001, 375, Table 9.2). Between 1975 and 1995, deaths from heart attacks plummeted in older age groups; more than a quarter of the decline has been attributed to aspirin use (Heidenreich & McClellan 2001, 384).

Drawing on this information, we can estimate how many people died unnecessarily because they didn't have this lifesaving information about aspirin in 1969. The numbers are large, because cardiovascular disease is the #1 killer in the United States. The 20-year gag order imposed on aspirin manufacturers cost approximately 1.7 million American lives (Heidenreich & McClellan 2001, 374, 376).[10]

> *Thus, aspirin has perhaps the best benefit-to-risk ratio of any proven therapy for acute MI [myocardial infarction or heart attack].*
> —American Heart Association, 1997

In about 25% of high-risk patients, aspirin also prevents ischemic stroke, which is caused by platelet clumping in narrowed blood vessels in the brain (Antiplatelet Trialists' Collaboration 1994, 81–106). Strokes and other forms of cerebrovascular disease are the third highest cause of death in the United States.

As it turns out, aspirin does more than prevent heart attacks and ischemic stroke. Aspirin may also be effective at preventing colorectal cancer (Algra & Rothwell 2012, 518–27; Rothwell, Price, Fowkes, et al. 2012, 1602–12; Rothwell, Wilson, Price, et al. 2012, 1591–601; Manzano & Pérez-Segura 2012, 327–41; Chan, Arber, Burn, et al. 2012, 164–78; Thun, Jacobs, & Patrono 2012, 259–67; Rothwell, Wilson, Elwin, et al. 2010, 1741–50) and other cancers (Rothwell, Wilson, Price, et al. 2012; Mills, Wu, Alberton, et al. 2012, 560–67).

Cancer is the number two killer in the United States. Had Americans taken aspirin for prevention of heart attacks in the 1970s instead of in the 1990s, aspirin's ability to prevent some cancers would have been known earlier. Aspirin, the humble over-the-counter pain reliever, affects the three major causes of disease-induced death in the industrialized world today.

Like all drugs, aspirin has side effects too. Chronic aspirin use increases the chance of hemorrhagic (as opposed to ischemic) strokes, which are caused by excessive bleeding in the brain, rather than platelet clumping. Stomach bleeding can occur as well. When considering daily aspirin use, both risks and benefits should be considered in consultation with a health care provider.

Ironically, if aspirin had to undergo the animal toxicology tests that the FDA demands today, this lifesaving drug probably would never have made it into human trials. Instead, it would have been left on the laboratory shelf when the company scientists saw the stomach ulcers in rats that had been treated with high doses of aspirin.

Some of aspirin's beneficial effects can probably be gained using diet and lifestyle alterations. For example, the Zone Diet, pioneered by Dr. Barry Sears (1995), was designed specifically to balance the eicosanoids to promote health. During the time that Sears was developing his dietary recommendations, he visited The Upjohn Company to glean information from our scientists, because Upjohn was a leader in the eicosanoid field.

Indeed, before the 1990s, Upjohn was the world's primary supplier of prostaglandins. University researchers simply had to tell us what they wanted to do and agree to send us reprints of their resulting publications to be gifted with hundreds—or even thousands—of dollars of prostaglandins of their choice. As the number of samples we gave out increased, publications on prostaglandins increased in parallel. Our scientists often showed a slide illustrating this relationship, which was an excellent example of research synergy between academia and industry.

Critics of the pharmaceutical industry are often concerned that companies build on university research. However, the exchange goes both ways. Universities often benefit from the production ability of pharmaceutical firms, which can give them drugs that would be prohibitive to purchase or make. If the proposed research is of special interest to a company, it might even provide money to execute the experiments.

As Amendment-driven regulatory demands have kept increasing, drug companies have had to put much more effort into development than into research. They increasingly rely on discoveries made and patented by universities to acquire NCEs for their pipeline. Without the Amendments, pharmaceutical firms would likely be devoting about 50% of their R&D budget to research, as they did in the early 1970s (Hansen 1979, 166; Schwartzman 1976, 70; Grawbowski 1976, 27; Schnee 1970, 220), instead of the 15% that they spend today (LaMattina 2013, 71).

Chapter 16

Off-Label Use Shows How the Market Can Determine Effectiveness

D octors who became aware of aspirin's beneficial effects in the 1960s and 1970s by reading medical journals, attending medical conventions, or talking to other physicians were able to use aspirin to prevent or treat heart attacks. However, most doctors were unaware of aspirin's benefits. Squibb and other drug firms probably knew more about aspirin than anyone else, but they couldn't share their knowledge for fear that the FDA would prosecute them for promoting off-label use.

... physicians who, due to FDA restraints, lack truthful off-label information may unwittingly cause harm to patients by denying them an effective treatment alternative.
—Jonathan Emord, lead counsel in several major legal initiatives against the FDA

A drug is approved by the FDA for marketing only for the indication or disease for which it was tested. For example, aspirin was a pain reliever. If any aspirin manufacturer mentioned its lifesaving benefits for heart attacks, the FDA could prosecute it for mislabeling its product, even if the information it shared was truthful. The FDA considers any such information misleading unless the agency has approved the new use after extensive clinical trials and has reviewed the language used to describe it.

Consequently, drug companies were forbidden to educate doctors and the public about aspirin's beneficial effects for almost 20 years. Doctors can legally prescribe aspirin or any drug to their patients, even for a different indication (disease) than its approved use, but drug companies are not allowed to share such off-label uses with the doctors. Off-label prescribing is so common that it accounts for between 20% and 60% of all prescriptions (Tabarrok 2000, 25–53; Conko 2011, 149–87, esp. 154). Off-label drug uses that are eventually approved by the FDA are usually common medical practice an average of 2.5 years earlier (Beales 1996, 281–305).

For example, when the FDA finally approved propranolol in 1968, it was for a relatively minor indication. Doctors who knew about propranolol's success in Europe for angina and hypertension could use it off-label to save their patients' lives until those indications were approved by the FDA in 1973 and 1976, respectively (Tabarrok 2000, 35). Doctors who weren't aware of the drug's broader applications didn't prescribe this lifesaving medication for patients who desperately needed it. Drug representatives from the companies selling propranolol would have gladly educated the physicians, but the FDA forbade their doing so.

Sometimes the FDA won't approve a drug because the FDA knows it's likely to be widely prescribed off-label. In the 1970s, the FDA declined to approve an anti-worm drug, levamisole, because of reports that it boosted immunity. Indeed, levamisole was so effective that it was approved in the 1990s for colon cancer (Tabarrok 2000, note 19). How many lives might have been saved had levamisole been approved for treatment of worms and prescribed off-label by oncologists aware of its immune-boosting properties? The FDA chose to check off regulatory boxes rather than putting a potentially lifesaving drug on the market 20 years earlier.

When I worked for Upjohn, the FDA forbade pharmaceutical salespeople (drug reps) from even bringing a physician's attention to studies that were published in medical journals and that described off-label uses for approved drugs. Consumer groups have challenged the FDA on the grounds that such prohibitions violate the constitutional guarantee of free speech. Although drug reps can now share published studies under certain conditions, the First Amendment issues have not been fully resolved (Conko 2011, 167–80). Meanwhile, the FDA aggressively prosecutes drug companies for providing physicians with information about off-label use, and it demands billions of dollars in settlements (Conko 2011, 163–64).

Arizona has enacted legislation that will allow pharmacists and drug reps to share truthful information with the state's doctors in spite of the FDA's prohibition on this practice (Maharrey 2017). Why did Arizona take such a drastic step?

To get FDA approval for adding a supplemental or new indication for a marketed drug, companies must do effectiveness or Phase 3 studies, which are the most-expensive and time-consuming part of any development program. In the early 1990s, the FDA took an average of 4 months longer to review those applications than it did for the original drug approval (DiMasi, Brown, & Lasagna 1996, 315–37). The FDA took 7 years to give acyclovir supplemental approval to treat the virus that causes shingles, a painful and reoccurring skin rash; the original application was approved in 10 months (Tabarrok 2000, 28).

Unfortunately, most doctors are so busy that they have little time to keep up with new research. Most of their knowledge about new medicines comes from meeting with drug reps, who keep physicians informed about new drugs and their FDA-approved uses. Consequently, two-thirds of surveyed neurologists, cardiologists, and oncologists believe that drug reps should be allowed to share data about off-label use with them. More than 60% of those doctors say that the FDA's policy of limiting off-label information makes it more difficult to learn about new uses for drugs and medical devices (Competitive Enterprise Institute 1995).

Frequently, the off-label uses for new drugs save more lives or alleviate more suffering than will the original indication for which the drug was approved. Aspirin is a prime example of such a drug. By suppressing information exchange about new uses for marketed drugs, the FDA condemns Americans to needless suffering and premature death.

Some critics of the pharmaceutical industry believe that no off-label use should be permitted until the FDA approves the supplemental indication. Because off-label use accounts for such a large percentage of prescriptions, both drug companies and the FDA would be completely overwhelmed in the attempt to comply. Very few applications would actually be submitted and make it through the approval process. Patients would be left to suffer and die as knowledge about marketed drugs that could have helped them is simply abandoned.

The FDA, even with cooperation from drug manufacturers, could not review drugs in its lengthy testing process at a pace equal to that at which physicians discover beneficial off-label use.
—William Christopher, Food and Drug Law Journal, 1993

Chapter 17

Development Costs Skyrocket

As the Amendments increased development time, thereby delaying the availability of new drugs and their off-label uses, the cost of development skyrocketed. While development times tripled, the costs of taking a drug from the lab bench to the marketplace soared even more.

When breakthrough drugs are discovered, several different companies are usually striving to get their version to the marketplace first. The company that succeeds in winning this race will usually enjoy the highest market share and profit the most (Bond & Lean 1977). The runners-up will make money too, but the amount will often be a mere fraction of what the first-to-market company gains.

However, all of the companies have usually put more than a decade into development before they know who will become the market leader and who will have a similar drug with a smaller market share. When the leading drug fails some patients, those people may find that the small differences in chemical structure in a me-too drug make a big difference in their clinical outcome.

Because being the first-to-market leader is so profitable, drug companies have great incentive to do whatever they can to compress the development timeline. Instead of doing sequential studies, they may choose to run them simultaneously. If the scientists aren't sure of the needed

Figure 2. Post-Amendment (black squares)[11] and Pre-Amendment (gray squares)[12] Average Out-of-Pocket R&D Costs per NCE Plotted against Median Year of NCE Approval.[13]

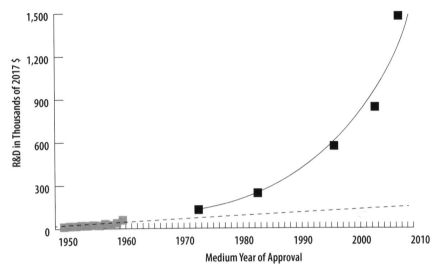

Medium Year of Approval

dose, they may run extra doses just to be sure that they won't have to repeat the animal study.

Consequently, we'd expect that tripling the development time would increase development costs by an even larger factor. As Figure 2 shows, that's exactly what happened after the passage of the Amendments. Costs increased exponentially and are still doing so, even though development time has leveled off, largely as a result of manufacturers' attempts to compress the development timeline.

Figure 2 illustrates the out-of-pocket R&D costs (actual expenditures) from the time an NCE is first made by company chemists until the FDA approves the drug for sale. Those costs don't include an adjustment for the time value of money or capitalization over the many years of development time. For post-Amendment studies, capitalizing out-of-pocket costs almost doubles the cost per NCE (Hansen 1979; DiMasi, Hansen, Grabowski, et al. 1991, 107–42; DiMasi, Hansen, & Grabowski 2003; DiMasi & Grabowski 2007, 469–79).

Those costs include the drugs that never make it to the marketplace because of safety problems, lack of effectiveness, or too few anticipated sales to make them worthwhile. More than 80% of the out-of-pocket cost of bringing a new drug to market is the cost of the failures leading up to an approved drug (Clymer 1970, 123–24). Most new drugs fail during development; those that finally make it to market are the exception rather than the rule.

Figure 2 uses post-Amendment development costs that are estimated by the same methodology for each time period. Even if one is skeptical about the exact costs generated by this methodology (Public Citizen 2001; Global Alliance for TB Drug Development 2001; DiMasi, Hansen, & Grabowski 2004), using a consistent way to calculate them allows us to be sure of whatever trend we find. The trend is pretty obvious: development costs are growing substantially every decade with no end in sight. If they continue unabated, they will become unsustainable, and we will have no new drugs at all.

… the estimates by DiMasi and colleagues of the cash outlays required to bring a new drug to market and the time profile of those costs provide a reasonably accurate picture of the mean R&D cash outlays for NCEs first tested in humans between 1970 and 1982.
—US Office of Technology Assessment, 1993

In attempting to replicate the results from DiMasi, Hansen, and Grabowski (2003), Adams and Brantner (2006, 420–28) came up with slightly higher estimates for the development costs of NCEs. Higher, lower, and similar estimates of NCE development costs have been reported by other investigators (Paul, Mytelka, Dunwiddie, et al. 2010, 203–14). The lower estimates usually result from the following: (a) disregarding the cost of failures (Ruwart 2005b, 24), (b) not including some of the clinical trials (DiMasi, Hansen, & Grabowski 2008, 319–24), and (c) diluting the estimates with approved drugs that are not NCEs (DiMasi, Hansen, & Grabowski 2004), such as different doses or changes in formulation.

The higher estimates sometimes include discovery costs leading up to the chemical design of an NCE (Gilbert, Henske, & Singh 2003, 1–10), not just costs accruing from the time the drug was first made or discovered.

The cost of getting FDA approval for an NCE increased post-Amendment much more rapidly than it had in the 1950s. Manufacturers spent 2.4 times as much to bring a new drug to market in 1968 than they had before Amendment passage (Baily 1972). Some drug companies were reporting a 10-fold increase in R&D costs per NCE in the early 1970s (Mund 1970, 125; Sarett 1974). Industry-wide data suggested an overall 8-fold increase in R&D per NCE between 1960–61 and 1970–74 (Grabowski Vernon, & Thomas 1978). Because the cost of developing NCEs goes up each year, the difference between pre-Amendment and post-Amendment developing costs goes up each year too.

The development costs illustrated in Figure 2 do not include the Phase 4 studies that are increasingly required by the FDA. From 1990 to 2010, US companies spent an average of $474 million (in 2015 dollars) in Phase 4 studies after FDA approval (DiMasi, Grabowski, & Hansen 2016).

Chapter 18

Regulatory Costs Determine What You Pay at the Pharmacy

A re rising pharmaceutical prices linked to the soaring R&D costs caused by the Amendments? To answer that question, we can compare the cost of an average branded (nongeneric) prescription drug with the capitalized R&D costs per NCE. Capitalized costs include the time value of the investment that companies make over the long years of development, and so they more accurately reflect the real cost of putting a new drug on the market.

Figure 3 shows how the average price of a branded prescription drug (that is, the pharmacy price of an NCE) rises along with soaring R&D costs. Indeed, almost all of the change in what we pay at the pharmacy for new drugs can be explained by the regulatory-driven increases in R&D per NCE ($r^2 = 0.94$ for the technically inclined).[14] The 1962 Amendments not only created delays in getting us lifesaving drugs but also created the high drug prices that so many decry.

Because the effects of the regulations are mostly unseen by outsiders, some critics of the pharmaceutical industry assume that greed is the driving force behind soaring pharmaceutical prices. As Figure 3 illustrates, the rising cost of getting FDA approval is the true culprit.

Figure 3. Inflation-Adjusted Average Branded Prescription Drug Price[15] as a Function of Pre-Amendment (black square)[16] and Post-Amendment (gray squares)[17] Capitalized New Drug R&D.

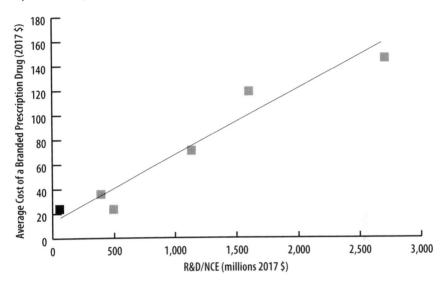

The soaring drug prices of the past several decades give the impression that they've always been on the rise. In fact, real (inflation-adjusted) drug prices *fell 32%* from 1949 to 1961. In the decade after the Amendments passed, drug prices fell only 2% (Telser 1975, 207–23, esp. 223). In the following decades, as development costs increased in response to the ever-growing regulatory demands of the Amendments, drug prices did too.

Some critics of the pharmaceutical industry fault the drug companies for putting so little into R&D. They don't seem to realize that drug companies put more of their sales dollars into R&D than virtually any other economic sector. Unfortunately, most of this money goes to meet regulatory demands rather than to discover new and better drugs.

For example, from 2000 to 2012, the drug companies spent an average of 18% of their sales dollars on R&D, more than any other manufacturing sector. The semiconductor industry spent 15%, followed by computer and electronics at 12% (Pham 2015, 13, Table 5). About 17% of all US research and development spending comes from the pharmaceutical industry (PhRMA 2016, 110).

> *Pharmaceutical firms invest as much as five times more in research and development, relative to their sales, than [does] the average US manufacturing firm.*
> —Congressional Budget Office, Research and Development
> in the Pharmaceutical Industry, 2006

Money that is not spent on R&D goes for advertising, manufacturing, payouts to investors, administration, and other miscellaneous expenditures. The Amendments have increased the costs of advertising, manufacturing, and return to investors as detailed next. If we were able to estimate the costs as we do for NCE development, we would likely find a similar relationship between those outlays and branded pharmaceutical prices as seen in Figure 3.

For example, the Amendments gave the FDA the power to seize all supplies of a manufactured drug if an advertisement did not meet the FDA's criteria (Jondrow 1972, 21–22). To avoid such seizures, manufacturers routinely submit their ads to the FDA before airing them.

The FDA almost always gives some sort of corrective feedback. The material is rewritten and resubmitted, and frequently it goes back and forth several times. Clearly, this process takes a great deal more time, effort, and money than simply putting together an unregulated advertisement.

The package insert, the detailed information that comes with every drug, goes through a process similar to the ads. However, because of its complexity and length, this review is much more time-consuming, intense, and fraught with disagreements over phraseology, specific warnings and restrictions, etc. What looks on paper like a simple advertising budget must account for all of the Amendment-driven costs.

Readers might legitimately ask, "Doesn't all this review make the advertising and package insert more accurate and understandable?" I simply invite readers to read the package inserts that come with each drug or to watch some of the television ads to answer that question. The long list of potential side effects that the FDA insists must follow every television commercial causes the listener to tune out and dismiss most of them as unlikely, thus reducing their value (Sivanathan & Kakkar 2017, 1-6). The detailed reviews are just one more delay in getting lifesaving drugs to market, as well as increasing their cost at the pharmacy. A better question to ask might be whether or not such costs give us comparable benefit.

The manufacturing process has also been greatly affected by Amendment-driven FDA oversight, as detailed in Chapter 12. Manufacturers not only must operate according to FDA procedures, but also must keep a considerable amount of documentation showing that they did so.

As regulations increase costs exponentially, fewer drugs are profitable. Only one out of eight drugs tested in people after 1992 made it to market, which is about half of the rate of the 1980s and early 1990s (DiMasi, Grabowski, & Hansen 2016; Hay, Thomas, Craighead, et al. 2014, 40-51; DiMasi, Reichert, Feldman, et al. 2013, 329-35; Paul, Mytelka, Dunwiddie, et al. 2010, 203-14). Only 20-30% of the new drugs that were approved made enough money to recover their R&D costs (Vernon, Golec, & DiMasi 2010, 1002-05). The best-selling 10% of drugs accounted for about 50% of sales (Grabowski, Vernon, & DiMasi 2002, 11-29, esp. 22-23, 27).

Consequently, pharmaceutical new drug development is becoming riskier, more costly, and ever more dependent on blockbuster drugs. To attract the capital necessary to develop a new drug, the industry—especially the smaller biotech companies—must promise higher rates of return to its investors. Why else would people put their money on the line for more than a decade when most of the drugs entering clinical testing fail after losing millions, if not billions, of dollars?

Chapter 19

What Would Drug Prices Have Been Without the Amendments?

B efore the Amendments, the price of bringing an NCE to market was increasing slowly over time. Although costs weren't calculated in exactly the same way as in post-Amendment studies, we can get a rough idea of how much money it would take to bring an NCE to market if pre-Amendment trends had continued.

To make this comparison, we can see that capitalized costs rather than out-of-pocket costs are appropriate. Post-Amendment new drugs took about three times as long to develop as did the pre-Amendment ones. Capitalized costs take into account the time value of money, which approximately doubles the out-of-pocket costs that a manufacturer invests over a 12-year to 14-year development time.

DiMasi, Grawbowski, and Hansen (2016) found that NCEs approved between 2005 and 2013 (average approval date 2008) cost an estimated $2,558 million (capitalized in 2013 dollars) to discover and develop. If we assume that pre-Amendment out-of-pocket costs would continue to increase as slowly as they did before Amendment passage, they would have been about $146 million (2013 dollars) in 2008. Capitalization would bring that sum to about $208 million (2013 dollars), using 10.1% as the cost of capital over a 4-year development time.[18] The figures suggest that the Amendments have increased development costs per NCE and their prices at the pharmacy about 12 times over what they would have otherwise been. However, other data suggest that the rough extrapolations may actually underestimate the negative impact of the Amendments.

For example, testosterone was approved in 1953, before Amendment passage (Androgel® 2007). Compounding pharmacies, which are able to make individualized specialty drugs, used to put together testosterone creams when doctors prescribed those formulations for their patients. The FDA prohibits pharmacies from advertising their compounded products to doctors. Such advertising would cause the FDA to reclassify compounded products as drugs that were required to go through the burdensome regulatory process.

However, doctors can ask compounding pharmacies to provide an off-patent drug such as testosterone on a per patient basis. Physicians used to prescribe those creams for men striving to retain youthful testosterone levels.

In 2011, the pharmaceutical firm, AbbVie, took its testosterone cream, Androgel®, through the FDA's post-Amendment regulatory process so that the company's sales reps could tell doctors how it helped to alleviate the symptoms of "male menopause" (andropause) (US FDA annual ed.). Androgel® initially cost 23 times more than the compounding pharmacies had been charging (Faloon 2011, 7).

The FDA forbids pharmacies to compound products that mimic marketed ones. Consequently, by 2016, a month's supply of testosterone cream, which would have cost about $50 per month through a compounding pharmacy, cost as much as $500 if purchased as Androgel® (Drug Watch n.d.).[19] This price stabilization, at about 10 times that of the compounded product, suggested that the post-Amendment regulatory demands resulted in price increases at the pharmacy of about a factor of 10.

Similarly, progesterone, which had also been marketed before passage of the Amendments, had been compounded as an injection to prevent premature births. Some women don't make enough of this crucial hormone to maintain their pregnancies. When KV Pharmaceutical took progesterone through the FDA's Orphan Drug process, which gave

Makena® a 7-year monopoly, the cost per injection went from $15–20 to $1,500 (Lowe 2011).

The Orphan Drug Act was a bandage put into place to counter some of the innovation loss (Chapters 21–24) caused by the Amendments. Companies refused to develop drugs when the patient population was too small to allow recovery of ever-increasing development costs. The 7-year monopoly gave companies the ability to charge whatever they wished so they would develop such orphans. As might be expected, those orphans became very pricey.

The public protested progesterone's price hike; the FDA announced that it wouldn't prosecute compounding pharmacies that still elected to provide injectable progesterone. KV Pharmaceutical then slashed Makena's price to $690 per injection, still about 34 times more than its compounded price. Because about 20 injections are needed per pregnancy, patient costs went from under $500 to more than $13,000 (Faloon 2011, 13).

Keep in mind that both testosterone and progesterone were older, generic drugs. Thus, a wealth of data was available to streamline studies necessary to satisfy the post-Amendment regulatory requirements. Companies knew how much drug to give, how often, and how to manufacture it. Success was virtually assured. No research was required to discover those drugs, a cost that was included in all of the estimates shown in Figure 2.

If KV and AbbVie had started with a typical NCE rather than drugs that were already marketed for decades, then their R&D costs—and consequently their pricing—would have been much higher. Both AbbVie and KV were able to streamline their clinical development program and to avoid costly mistakes because of the wealth of information available for the two drugs. Without such knowledge and experience, their development costs—and their prices at the pharmacy— would have *at least* doubled. In other words, the drugs would have cost 20 times or 68 times as much as their compounded counterparts had they been new NCEs.

Compounding is an expensive process relative to the mass production that most pharmaceuticals undergo, because the pharmacist prepares each prescription individually. Thus, the compounding cost of testosterone and injectable progesterone is at *least* two-fold higher than it would be when those two drugs are manufactured on an assembly line.

Consequently, AbbVie and KV enjoyed *at least* a two-fold saving when they mass produced Androgel® and Makena® instead of compounding them. Consequently, the real pricing differential at the pharmacy between pre-Amendment and post-Amendment drugs undergoing standard manufacturing is probably *at least* 40 times for Androgel and 136 times for Makena.

Such back-of-the-envelope estimations suggest that the average branded drug costs about 40 times more because of the Amendments. Put another way, a drug that costs $400 today after going through the post-Amendment regulatory process would probably cost a mere $10 in the absence of the Amendments. The Orphan Drug Act increased pricing for drugs developed under its umbrella another 3.4 times.

Even those estimated increases in drug prices that have been caused by the Amendments are probably conservative. In a consistent regulatory environment, rather than one in which the FDA's demands increase every year, R&D costs per NCE might have stabilized or even gone down. Today's R&D has become ever more streamlined because of innovations in the way research is conducted, but it has been outpaced by increasing regulatory requirements.

For example, in the 1960s, researchers still had to make many of the compounds that they used in their experiments themselves, especially radioactive ones. Scientists had to spend a few days or even a few weeks of time preparing the products they wanted to use as part of their tests.

Imagine the cost in time and money if you had to grind your own flour, grow your own yeast cultures, and cut firewood for your oven so you could make bread! The difference between today and yesterday is immense: today, you simply go to the grocery store and choose from a variety of products.

Similarly, scientists today can order a vast array of chemicals, even radio-active ones, instead of making their own ingredients for their experiments. The saving in time and money is comparable to the difference between buy-ing bread and making it—along with *all* of its components—from scratch.

Today, many research tests are automated. Hundreds, if not thou-sands, of potential drugs can be checked for the desired activity in days or weeks. Before we had robotics to do the tests, evaluating that number of chemicals could take months or even years.

We now understand more about how our bodies work than we once did. Instead of dosing animals to see the effects we want, we can use a surrogate test instead. If we know the critical component (e.g., enzyme or gene) we are trying to affect, we can isolate it in a test tube and run hun-dreds of tests instead of conducting a couple of dozen tests in animals, which take much longer and are more expensive in both time and money.

Today, we use computers to analyze our data in minutes. I remember us-ing slide rules and early calculators, which required hours—or even days—for statistical analyses. Those computations are now virtually instantaneous.

Just as research has become more efficient, drug development would have too, if not for continually increasing regulatory demands. As mentioned earlier, companies have strong incentives to compress the development time-line to be first to market. The 4 years that it took before the Amendments to get a drug from the lab bench to the marketplace might have been main-tained or even further compressed without any compromise in safety.

We can simply speculate what might have been. However, the in-creased costs of injectable progesterone and testosterone cream before and after going through FDA's formal development process suggest that the Amendments have probably increased new NCE R&D by at least 40 times over what they otherwise would have been.

The Orphan Drug Act, one of the legislative bandages that were put into place to stop the innovation losses caused by the Amendments, only increased drug prices further by granting the drugs a 7-year monopoly. However, as the next chapter illustrates, the Amendments have routinely created monopolies even without the Orphan Drug Act.

Chapter 20

How Have the Amendments Enabled the Greedy?

O nce a new drug's patent expires, generic manufacturers must go through an Abbreviated New Drug Application (ANDA) before they can market it. The FDA requires bioequivalence studies that take about 2 years and about $5 million to complete (Faloon 2011, 139; Faloon 2017, 7–12, esp. 9). Those studies must demonstrate that the generic drug is absorbed into the blood stream at the same rate as the branded drug.

However, the FDA takes an additional 3.5 years to review the new studies and approve the marketing of the new generic drug (Barlas 2014, 833, 843–45). In other words, the FDA can take longer to review a new generic drug application than the agency took to examine the truck-load of data submitted when the same drug was first approved. Review times are, on average, longer than the generic company takes to run the FDA-mandated studies.

The rising cost—in time and money—of getting a generic drug to market is limiting the number of suppliers. Prices for generics have increased sharply over the past several years as a result (Fein 2014). For some generics, supplies have become dangerously limited, because the FDA imposes more and more regulatory restrictions on the manufacturers (Fein 2014; Forbes 2015).

As regulatory demands increase on generic manufacturing, companies that produce the older generics find them unprofitable. This finding is especially true for companies that don't raise prices much on older drugs. Eventually, companies shut down production until only one manufacturer remains. This reality creates an environment ripe for exploitation.

DARAPRIM

The older generics are often bought or licensed from the sole manufacturer by a small company whose only intention is to greatly increase the price. Daraprim, for example, is used to treat toxoplasmosis in fewer than 13,000 Americans annually. Many are AIDS patients, who are more susceptible than the rest of the population to this type of infection. They generally take daraprim along with sulfadiazine.

In 2014, Turing Pharmaceuticals bought daraprim from Impax, the only manufacturer still supplying the drug in the United States. GlaxoSmithKline had introduced daraprim in 1953. Its price was a mere $1 per pill until Glaxo sold the marketing rights to CorePharma in 2010. Core was acquired by Impax in 2014.

Shortly after acquiring daraprim, Turing's CEO, Martin Shkreli, announced his plan to increase its price from $13.50, the Impax price, to $750 a pill (Pollack 2015). Turing attempted to keep its monopoly by using a closed distribution system to prevent other generic companies from getting enough daraprim to do the comparative studies required by the FDA (Lowe 2014). Of course, even if daraprim had been made available to other generic companies, the FDA-required studies to market this off-patent drug would still take years. In the meantime, Turing could set the price. When regulations stop or delay competition, price gouging is made easy.

Glaxo, the large pharmaceutical firm that developed daraprim, was content with supplying this generic drug at an affordable price for many years. Today, small drug firms that don't want to do the hard work of R&D are actively seeking generics that serve a needy population and have only one supplier (Lowe 2015). If a drug company can gain exclusive marketing rights, the patients who need that generic are at its mercy, courtesy of a regulatory environment that drives competitors out of business.

EPI-PEN

As allergies to peanuts, eggs, and other foodstuffs increase, the Epi-Pen has become a common fixture in many households and schools. A severe allergic reaction can cause the airway to swell, making breathing difficult and, in some cases, becoming life-threatening. The Epi-Pen can be used to self-inject with a dose of epinephrine, which quickly restores breathing ability.

The Epi-Pen is used frequently to save the lives of children and adults who inadvertently eat allergens or are allergic to bee stings. In 2007, the Epi-Pen was selling for $57. By 2016, Epi-Pens, which expire after a year on the shelf, were sold only in packages of two. The retail price was touted as $600 (Willingham 2016). I was actually quoted a whopping $800 at my pharmacy.

Mylan, which acquired the Epi-Pen in 2007, was able to raise its prices once Mylan became the only seller. In late 2015, Sanofi withdrew Auvi-Q, Epi-Pen's last true competitor, from the market after some suspected device malfunctions (Stanton 2016). Teva had submitted an application for a generic version of the Epi-Pen to the FDA. However, the agency felt "certain major deficiencies" needed to be addressed (Helfand 2016a).

Adamis wanted to market a syringe prefilled with epinephrine, the active drug in the Epi-Pen. Some diabetics must inject themselves with insulin, so use of a syringe—rather than an Epi-Pen-like device—is not unprecedented. The FDA demanded more studies, however (Helfand 2016b). Mylan's monopoly was due to the excessive regulations that the Amendments have engendered.

Luckily for consumers, Auvi-Q re-entered the market in early 2017. In the last half of 2016, the generic autoinjector Adrenaclick® was approved. Savvy consumers now have lower-priced alternatives. Mylan has started giving coupons with substantial discounts for Epi-Pen in an attempt to keep its market share.

Some people are under the impression that a drug company can charge anything it wants. What stops the companies is the fear that their competition will undersell them and take their customers; after all, who wants to pay more than they have to for expensive drugs? The Amendments, by limiting and sometimes eliminating competition, have actually made price gouging easier.

Chapter 21

Innovation Is Imperative

S o far, we've seen how the delays in getting lifesaving drugs to market and information to physicians have resulted in premature deaths of millions of Americans. We've seen how the Amendments have created soaring pharmaceutical prices by increasing development costs and destroying competition. Even more deadly and costly, however, are the loss of innovations caused by the Amendments.

When drug companies spend ever-increasing amounts of money to satisfy FDA regulations, they have fewer resources to devote to innovation. No matter how wealthy people are, they can't buy cures that have not yet been discovered. In 1836, Nathan Rothschild, who was one of the wealthiest men in the world, died needlessly of an infection because antibiotics had not yet been discovered (Rothschild n.d.).

Loss of innovation is, quite literally, a matter of life and death. In the early 20th century, the primary cause of death was infection; the 1918 flu epidemic alone killed about 4% of the world's population (1918 Flu Pandemic n.d., note 3). Pneumonia and flu were the leading cause of death in the early 20th century, followed by tuberculosis and gastrointestinal infections, which often led to ulceration. In 1900, those diseases were responsible for about 30% of all deaths in the United States (Centers for Disease Control n.d.).

All that changed with better sanitation, wider availability of refrigerated trucking that allowed off-season fruits and vegetables to be trans-
ported, large-scale production of vitamins, and discovery of antibiotics.
The survival rate for severe pneumonia went from 15% in the early 20th
century to 90% toward the end of it (Austrian & Gold 1964, 759–76). Pneumonia and flu dropped from the first to the sixth leading cause of death in
the United States (CDC n.d.). Overall, death from infectious disease in the
United States dropped 95% from 1900 to 1980 (Armstrong, Conn, & Pinner 1999, 61–66). Individuals who would have died from infections were
quite literally brought back from the brink of death by antibiotics.

The almost miraculous turnaround led to those pharmaceuticals being labeled "wonder drugs" (Herrell 1943, 65–76, esp. p. 71). In 1969, the
US Surgeon General, Dr. William Stewart, is reputed to have said, "It is
time to close the book on Infectious Disease and declare the war against
pestilence won" (Spellberg 2009, 33). Indeed, during the last half of the
20th century, the developed world came to believe that only the weak,
frail, or elderly would ever succumb to this age-old scourge.

But times have changed. Young, healthy athletes are coming down
with infections after skinning their hands and knees sliding on artificial
turf (Lindenmayer, Schoenfeld, O'Grady, et al. 1998, 895–99). Within days,
a simple skin infection becomes blood borne and starts shutting down vital
organs. The very antibiotics that were hailed as wonder drugs are powerless
against these superbugs. Our children are once again at risk.

What are superbugs? They are the very bacteria that used to succumb
to our wonder drugs—except for one very important difference: they
have developed resistance to just about every drug in our pharmaceutical arsenal. An example is commonly called MRSA, or methicillin-resistant *Staphylococcus aureus*. Such superbugs have become a serious health
problem (Spellberg 2009).

MRSA started out in hospitals among the sick, who are usually more
susceptible to infection. MRSA was fought with antibiotics until the superbugs became resistant to just about any antibiotic that we could throw
at them. From the hospitals, those superbugs have migrated into nursing

homes, into the population at large, and finally into our gyms and other places where people are in close quarters and likely to have skin abrasions. At this time, most researchers believe that we need to keep finding new classes of antibiotics to counteract the threat of MRSA and other superbugs.

Even though cardiovascular disease is the primary killer in the United States and developed countries, infection is still number one worldwide because of its prevalence in developing countries (LaMattina 2013, 66). Even in the United States, an estimated 300,000 still succumb to infection each year (Spellberg 2009, 35).

Pharmaceutical firms are putting a great deal of money into the discovery and development of drugs to control the HIV virus but very little into developing new antibiotics. Between 1983 and 1987, the FDA approved 16 new antibiotics. Between 2003 and 2007, it approved only 5 (Spellberg 2009, 88). The number of major pharmaceutical companies trying to come up with new antibiotics has dropped during this time from 20 in 1993 to 2 in 2013 (LaMattina 2013, 66).

Why are companies rushing to develop drugs to thwart HIV but not MRSA and other resistant strains? After all, both infections kill most of their victims. The difference is that AIDS patients will be on drug therapy for their lifetime, while MRSA patients can be cured with short-term treatment. The high cost of development makes it extremely difficult for companies to recover their costs with a drug to be used for a week or two rather than for years. A company that does not recover development costs will eventually cease to exist.

Consequently, research is not undertaken in areas where recovery of development costs is not possible. In my early years at Upjohn, we focused less on development costs and more on the expertise we had to save lives. In later years, management cautioned us to consider carefully whether or not we could make back our ever-rising development costs before undertaking new projects.

When I joined Upjohn in 1976, it was still smarting from the economic loss of Panalba. The Infectious Disease Unit, once one of the company's proud leaders, gradually dwindled down to a handful of scientists as development costs rose.

The government is schizophrenic about antibiotics. After the Amendments made developing new antibiotics almost cost prohibitive, Congress tried to create new incentives for antibiotic development by adding 5 years to the patent life of designated new anti-infectives in 2012 (Pew Charitable Trusts 2013). However, such bandages are unlikely to entice many manufacturers into investing heavily in drugs that are designed for short-term use. The government's threat to permit generic competition of the antibiotic Cipro years before the patent expired (Associated Press 2001) makes manufacturers wary of any promises that bureaucrats might make.

The government wanted to stockpile Cipro in case of an emergency, but it didn't want to pay the price Bayer was charging. In 2001 when anthrax was sent through the mail to two senators and several media offices, Cipro was the only antibiotic approved for anthrax treatment (Jenkins 2001, A23). Other antibiotics worked against anthrax too, but because they hadn't gotten FDA approval for that particular disease, they couldn't be marketed for it (Abelson & Pollack 2001, B8). The government's threat to Cipro's patent status forced Bayer to lower its prices. The government got a short-term gain, but the long-term cost was to discourage antibiotic development even further.

Without innovations in antibiotics, humankind might very well fall prey to pestilence once again. Indeed, about 25% of the worldwide death toll is still due to bacterial and viral infections. A superbug that is resistant to all known antibiotics could spread rapidly in today's small world. Because very little research is currently in place, finding drugs worth developing could take longer than usual. By that time, millions more may pay the ultimate price for the Amendments.

Are there inexpensive herbs and other over-the-counter products that are useful against infections from bacteria, viruses, and parasites? Certainly! However, as we will explore in Chapters 33–35, doctors are largely unaware of them. Sellers of those products cannot legally promote them for infection unless they go through the expensive and time-consuming regulatory process that was spawned by the Amendments.

Chapter 22

The Amendments Slashed Innovation by Pharmaceutical Firms

n 1962, pharmaceutical firms were re-investing about 8% of their sales dollar into R&D. Over the next two decades, this percentage dropped steadily, until—by 1979—a mere 6.5% of sales revenue was put toward R&D (Grabowski, Vernon, & DiMasi 2002, 25). A 19% decrease in R&D might not seem like much, but it was coupled to another significant side effect of the Amendments: only 1 out of 10 (new molecular entities) recovered their development costs in the first decade after the Amendments passed (Grawbowski 1976, 37). Without cost recovery, money couldn't be put into research. Even though NCEs accounted for 20% of sales before the Amendments, between 1967 and 1971, NCEs contributed a mere 5.5% (Grawbowski 1976, 57).

Universities, funded by the government via grants, tried to fill the gap. However, because their discoveries couldn't be patented in the first couple of decades after the Amendments passed, no drug company would develop them. Taxpayer-funded discoveries were meant to belong to the people, but the Amendments had made patents necessary. Consequently, because universities were not equipped for drug development, those innovations languished on the laboratory shelves.

In 1980, Congress attempted to fix this problem by passing the Bayh-Dole Act, which allowed universities to patent their discoveries. They could then license the discoveries to pharmaceutical firms for development. Encouraged by the possibility of more NCEs, drug companies increased the percentage of their sales dollars that went into R&D. They became development agents for university-based discoveries, because the cost—in time, money, and regulatory know-how—of taking a new drug to market was beyond the scope of virtually all academic institutions.

In the 15 years after the passage of the Bayh-Dole Act, the percentage of the pharmaceutical sales dollar rose steadily each year until R&D had almost doubled (Grabowski, Vernon, & DiMasi 2002, 25). By 2013, 23% of sales went into R&D (PhRMA 2015, 66). However, most of this increase was used to meet the ever-increasing regulatory demands, rather than research to discover new NMEs.

When the Amendments were passed, about half of pharmaceutical R&D went to finding new medicines (Hansen 1979, 166; Schwartzman 1976, 70; Grabowski 1976, 27; Schnee 1970, 220). Today, only about 15% is devoted to innovation (LaMattina 2013, 71). The pharmaceutical companies spend so much on development that little is left for research.

Critics of the pharmaceutical industry complain that many of today's new drugs came originally from tax-supported universities. The Amendments were largely responsible for this shift by sacrificing research to development.

Chapter 23

Innovation Is Thwarted by the Amendments

B y requiring proof of effectiveness, the Amendments discouraged manufacturers from trying to develop truly novel, breakthrough drugs. For example, my own work on prostaglandins and liver disease came to the attention of a prominent FDA examiner, who took the time to call me personally. "Dr. Ruwart," he said, "I understand that you've filed a patent for the use of prostaglandins in liver disease. I want to encourage you and your company to develop this treatment for fibrotic liver disease. As you know, over 100,000 people die each year from liver failure; we simply don't have effective treatment for it."

The liver often scars when continuously exposed to a toxin such as the hepatitis virus or alcohol. We call that scarring "fibrosis." When fibrosis replaces enough of the liver, the organ can no longer do its job. The patient dies from liver failure.

The FDA examiner's call gave us hope that we could develop a prostaglandin for liver disease. Upjohn had invested many years and large sums of money in those potent, natural hormones. A treatment for chronic liver disease would save thousands, perhaps tens of thousands, of lives each year. For taking the risk of bringing such a novel drug to the market, Upjohn would reap the just reward of profit.

Unfortunately, even with the support of the FDA, development was not that easy. We would be the first to show that a drug could cure fibrotic liver disease. Consequently, we had no model to follow in designing the clinical trials that the FDA required. We did not know how many people needed to be in our study to meet the FDA's standard of statistical significance. We did not know how many years people would have to take our drug. We didn't know how much drug to use or how many years it would take for the fibrosis to heal. We didn't know how to easily track the disease with blood measurements or whether the FDA would even accept such a surrogate marker. Would we have to take biopsies, which required removing a piece of the liver from each patient, to watch the fibrosis disappear? Since the fibrosis was not necessarily uniform, how many pieces would we need to take? How often would we need to take them?

All of those uncertainties, which are common ones for the most innovative and novel drugs, made it unlikely that the first human effectiveness study would have the statistical significance required by the FDA. Consequently, if we didn't guess right on most of those parameters the first time, we would have to start over again.

Because we anticipated that this study would take several years, it became clear that the patent on our prostaglandin would probably run out before we received FDA approval unless we were able to design our study perfectly the first time. Our prostaglandin would go generic immediately, and we would be unable to recover our development costs. The decision not to develop a novel therapy for an untreatable and deadly disease was made, at least in part, because of conditions imposed by the 1962 Amendments.

Before 1962, Upjohn might have been able to market a prostaglandin for liver disease if the doctors who were given samples felt that their patients had improved. Indeed, doctors in other countries reported that treatment with Upjohn's natural products, PGE1 and PGE2, resolved hepatic failure—which usually leads to death—in subjects with viral hepatitis (Hyman, Yim, Krajden, et al. 1999, 329–36; Reus, Priego, Boix, et al. 1998, 84–86; Hemming, Cattral, Greig, et al. 1996, 177–85; Greig,

Cameron, Phillips, et al. 1994, 183–92; Sinclair & Levy 1991, 791–800; Sinclair, Greig, Blendis, et al. 1989, 1063–69; Bojić, Begović, Mijuskovi, et al. 1995, 471–75; Lim, Kwon, Lee, et al. 2006, 928–32).

Almost a decade after the decision to abandon development of a prostaglandin for liver disease, US studies with a prostaglandin chemically modified to stay in the body longer than the natural ones, showed promise in viral hepatitis patients as well (Flisiak & Prokopowicz 2000, 161–65; Flisiak & Prokopowicz 1997, 1419–25).

Unfortunately, the company that reported those confirmatory results couldn't market their prostaglandin for liver disease without jumping through the FDA's elaborate hoops for the new indication and licensing the Upjohn patent for prostaglandins in liver disease. By the time their prostaglandin was approved for liver disease, their patent on the modified prostaglandin would likely have expired, and they would not recover their development costs. Consequently, they didn't pursue development either.

Chapter 24

The Amendments Have Destroyed About 80% of Our Innovations

H ow many innovative, potentially lifesaving drugs never make it to the marketplace because of the added costs in time and money imposed by the Amendments? No one knows for sure, but the studies that have been done imply that we've lost about 80% of the innovations that we would have had in the absence of the Amendments.

Shortly after the Amendments passed, researchers began showing that pharmaceutical innovation had plummeted. Steven Wiggins (1981, 615–19) at Texas A&M University, for example, studied the relationship between regulatory stringency, measured by FDA approval times, and NCE approvals for the years 1968 through 1976. Even for those early post-Amendment years, when development costs were lower than they are now, he estimated an overall innovation loss of 52% caused by the Amendments.

Some disease classes lost more innovation than others did. New drugs for heart disease were reduced by an incredible 81%. This is a devastating finding, especially because heart disease is the biggest killer of both men and women in the United States.

Wiggins also examined innovation losses on the basis of the FDA's own ranking of a new drug's importance. Class A drugs provide an important therapeutic advance, class B drugs have a modest effect, and class

C drugs have a minimal one. He found a 54% decrease in class A innovations, a 39% reduction in B drugs, and a 38% decrease in C drugs.

Of course, we don't often know which drugs are most important, because drugs developed for one disease may eventually save more lives when used in another. Aspirin, originally marketed to alleviate pain, is saving lives today because of its beneficial effects in heart disease, which is the number one killer in the developed world.

The prostaglandin and liver disease example is a good illustration of why innovative drugs are less likely to be brought to market in the post-Amendment environment. A breakthrough drug comes with uncertainties concerning safety, dosing, measures of effectiveness, etc. More studies will have to be done to resolve such issues. The risk of failure is higher and the cost, as we've seen earlier, keeps skyrocketing.

Nevertheless, about 78% of the drugs entering Phase 1 in the United States in the past few decades have been "first-in-class" drug candidates. By the time that the FDA approves those products, only half of them have this designation. Truly new drugs have a harder time making it through the regulatory process than "me-too" drugs that are small improvements on older compounds (Long & Works 2013, 11). We know more about those older drugs, so we can more easily design studies that are likely to give the statistical significance that the FDA requires the first time around.

Before the Amendments, manufacturers could try to develop novel (and thus more risky) drugs more often, because the development costs were much lower than after the Amendments passed. Today, it often makes more economic sense to follow in the footsteps of pharmaceutical pioneers with a me-too drug, rather than to innovate.

Wiggins wasn't the only researcher to point to the devastating losses in innovation that followed the passage of the Amendments. Peltzman (1973, 1049–91) created a model that predicted pharmaceutical innovation quite accurately between 1948 and 1962 (Figure 4). Between the passage of the Amendments and 1972, actual innovation—measured by the number of NCE approvals—plummeted to less than half of what it otherwise would have been. Peltzman's findings are consistent with the findings of Wiggins.

Figure 4: Actual and Modeled Pre- and Post-Amendment Drug Innovations (NCEs vs. Year of Approval)[20]

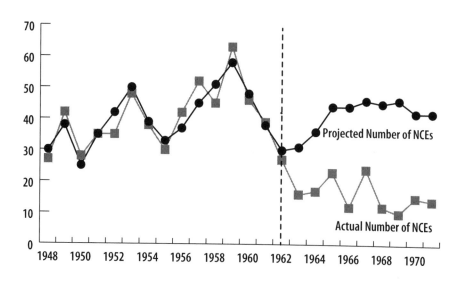

Investigators at Tufts University reported even more devastating findings: a 61% reduction in the number of NCEs between 1963 and 1972 and an incredible 81% reduction between 1975 and 1979 in the number of NCEs entering clinical trials. They also pointed out that the "4 years of Congressional hearings that attacked the pharmaceutical industry, its products, and its advertising and pricing policies" that preceded the passage of the Amendments slowed the FDA's willingness to approve NCEs and the manufacturers' willingness to invest in them (May, Wardell, & Lasagna 1983, 691–700). In 1974, the American Medical Association's House of Delegates voted to work for the repeal of the Amendments because new drugs had so much difficulty reaching the market (Wardell & Lasagna 1975, 15–16). Unfortunately, the Amendments remained in place and continue to thwart innovation.

Another Tufts' study (DiMasi 2001b, 301, Table I) found that 86 of the NCEs that had entered clinical testing between 1981 and 1992 had been approved by the time this study ended. Another 43 were still in testing; 8–13 of those might have eventually made it to the market according to the actual approval rate. In other words, as many as 99 NCEs might have ultimately been approved.

Before 1962, the rate of new chemical introductions in the United States was a little less than one-half the worldwide rate. In the decade following, the US rate dropped to little more than one-fifth the worldwide rate.
—David Schwartzman, economics professor at the New School for Social Research, New York, NY

Another 109 tests, however, had been abandoned by their manufacturer about halfway through their human testing (DiMasi 2001b, 305, Table II). Their problem wasn't safety or effectiveness; the tests simply weren't economically viable because "the commercial market [was] too limited" or the drugs were expected to give an "insufficient return on investment" (DiMasi 2001b, 304). More drugs were abandoned by their manufacturers in this study than were approved or expected to be approved. This finding suggests that the high development costs imposed by the Amendments cost us more than half of the new drugs that enter human testing!

Why didn't the pharmaceutical companies abandon the drugs before starting development, as Upjohn abandoned prostaglandins for liver disease? Unfortunately, because of the long development time and the increasing demands of the FDA virtually every year, it's almost impossible to predict what the costs will actually be. Consequently, many drugs are abandoned late in the development process when the company finally realizes that those drugs are financial losers. Unfortunately, the drugs might have been winners from the perspective of patients needing treatment for their disease, but the Amendments made them economically impractical. The ever-rising costs of development ensure that more and more potentially lifesaving drugs will be abandoned.

Without the Amendments creating skyrocketing development costs, we would not have lost so many of our innovations. If more than half of our new drugs are abandoned in late development, the 81% loss of innovation reported by Tufts for the 1970s might actually be an under-estimate. After all, development costs have skyrocketed since then, so we would expect even more potentially lifesaving drugs to be abandoned before they even reach human trials. Such a large innovation loss suggests that we might have five times as many new drugs today if it weren't for the Amendments.

One might legitimately ask if we truly need five times as many drugs as we have today. Obviously, the answer depends on whether the lost innovations are of significant medical value. Chapter 26 suggests that even if the lost innovations are only 25% as effective as the ones that we have now, the loss of life will far exceed that experienced by the United States from Amendment-driven delays in taking new drugs to market.

Chapter 25

Britain Does It Better

The FDA did not seem troubled by the loss of innovation that followed implementation of the Amendments. Initially, officials felt that fewer drugs were being approved because ineffective ones were being kept off the market. As we'll learn in Chapter 30, less than 10% of drugs marketed before passage of the Amendments were found to be ineffective, so the 50–80% loss in innovation was unlikely to be due to ensuring that only drugs that worked were approved.

FDA Commissioner Alexander Schmidt then shrugged off the loss of innovation as a result of drug companies having already picked "the low-hanging fruit" of research opportunities. Consequently, he reasoned, fewer drugs were left to develop. He noted that—after passage of the Amendments—there was a worldwide decline in new drugs, and he felt that finding supported his position (Schwartzman 1975b, 19). However, this explanation is not consistent with the facts.

Although innovation in the United States dropped precipitously after passage of the Amendments, the number of British discoveries did not (Grabowski, Vernon, & Thomas 1978, 147). Had the low-hanging fruit theory been correct, we would have expected both countries to experience a substantial decline in innovation, but British scientists continued to come up with new drugs at the same rate they had before Amendment passage.

However, the number of made-in-America drugs marketed in Britain fell just as they had in the United States. Innovation that didn't happen in the United States couldn't enter the British market. About half of drug discovery in the 1960s and 1970s was happening in the United States (Grabowski 1980; Temin 1980, 44), so less innovation there meant fewer lifesaving drugs introduced worldwide. Between 1967 and 1971, only 15% of new drugs in Britain came from the United States. Before the Amendments, 54% did (Grabowski 1976, 60).

In addition, most of the new drugs invented in the United States were marketed first in Europe (Pierce 1995). We tested new drugs there first because the regulatory pathways overseas were faster and less expensive. Consequently, Europeans had twice as many drugs in their pharmacies as Americans had (Wardell & Lasagna 1975, 57–59; Peltzman 1974, 13–18)!

Chapter 26

Innovators Lose Even When They Succeed

R egulatory demands that are costly in time and money fall heaviest on small, entrepreneurial biotech companies that are attempting to bring their innovations to the marketplace. Dendron Pharmaceuticals, for example, developed Provenge, a novel personalized treatment for prostate cancer patients. Immune cells are taken from the blood and "trained" in a test tube to attack the cancer cells. When put back into the bloodstream, those activated immune cells find and destroy the tumor. In the early 1990s, when Dendron's founder was running the initial tests, the FDA didn't regulate this type of cellular therapy (Centeno 2012), which was considered to be a form of medical practice, not a new pharmaceutical product.

Cancer patients treated with Provenge showed decreases in PSA, a blood marker often used to access disease status, as early as 1999 (Burch, Breen, Buckner, et al. 2000, 2175–82). The prostate cancer community began lobbying for FDA approval of Provenge, because—by then—the agency was firmly entrenched as a regulator of cellular therapy.

We know that it works, and we know why it works. In any rational regulatory environment, that would be reason to speed Provenge to market.
—*Wall Street Journal* editorial, "New Cancer Drugs," January 26, 2004

By late 2005, another study (Small, Schellhammer, Higano, et al. 2006, 3089–94) had demonstrated that 34% of the Provenge patients were still alive compared to 11% in the placebo group after 3 years of treatment. Drawing on those and subsequent trials, Drendron filed for FDA approval in 2006.

In March 2007, the FDA's Advisory Committee—composed of outside consultants—voted to approve Provenge. In May, however, the FDA decided that more studies were needed. It argued that even though survival was better in Provenge-treated patients, the time to disease progression, which had originally been designated as the study's main endpoint, wasn't statistically significant (Liu, Bross, & Whitten 2007). Although improved survival had not been expected, living longer was clearly the desired—and statistically significant—endpoint.

In retrospect, the physicians who conducted the study believed that the time to disease progression was probably a poor endpoint to use. Provenge took longer to act than did standard chemotherapies, because several weeks were probably necessary for it to invoke the maximum immune system response. The disease might have progressed somewhat before the full effect of the treatment was realized, and then it slowed precipitously as the body's own defenses attacked the cancer (Small, Schellhammer, Higano, et al. 2006).

Truly novel drugs, as Provenge was, act differently than expected sometimes, making the design of statistically significant studies challenging. Provenge actually performed better than expected, on the basis of survival rates, but the FDA wasn't willing to accept those results because the drug didn't affect time to disease progression, a standard parameter for chemotherapies that act in an entirely different way.

The FDA's refusal to approve this lifesaving drug in 2007 resulted in protests, death threats to two members of the advisory committee who had voted against it, lawsuits by patient support groups, and even congressional threats to investigate the FDA (Faloon 2011, 79–80; Roan 2007; Stein 2007). The FDA, however, did not relent.

In 2009, Dendreon reported on the additional studies mandated by the FDA; those studies were similar to the ones the company had submitted in 2006 (*Urology Times* 2009). On April 29, 2010, the FDA finally approved Provenge, but only for *advanced* prostate cancer (US FDA 2010a). Because of this restriction, insurance companies usually won't pay for Provenge treatment at earlier stages, where it is likely to be more effective.

The extra studies demanded by the FDA and the restrictions on the use had heavy costs in money, time, and lives. Provenge was initially priced at $93,000. The manufacturer needed to cover the costs of the extra FDA-mandated studies that simply confirmed what was already known. Had the FDA approved the drug when Provenge was first shown to decrease the surrogate marker PSA, the cost to the company and the patients would have been much lower. One doctor estimated that Provenge would have cost somewhere between $8,000 and $15,000, or about 10–15% as much, if it had remained unregulated by the FDA, as some other cellular procedures (such as in vitro fertilization) are (Centeno 2012, 17).

When my brother was diagnosed with late stage prostate cancer, his doctor offered him Provenge and told him that it might add 4.5 months to his life, according to the 2006 study (Small, Schellhammer, Higano, et al. 2006). Although 4.5 months was the median survival difference between the placebo and treatment group, the fact that three times as many treated patients were alive 3 years later suggests that some people responded very well to treatment, while others hardly benefited. Responders could expect to add years to their survival, while nonresponders would gain little or nothing.

Focusing on the group response, as the FDA prefers, rather than on the individual response causes us to miss the important finding that Provenge dramatically increases survival in certain individuals. Recognizing this finding, the National Cancer Institute, a division of the National Institutes of Health, is reviewing data from cancer treatment studies to see if small populations of patients, such as those responding to Provenge, had an exceptional response (NCI Staff 2017). If so, maybe we can identify the people most likely to benefit from a particular treatment before it's administered.

Many cancer treatments have serious side effects. Provenge was much better tolerated, because it basically consisted of the patient's own cells. However, as a result of the FDA's continued demands and its approval for advanced cancer patients only, Dendreon had to file for bankruptcy (Brickley & Winslow 2014). Thus, it was eventually bought out by Valeant Pharmaceuticals International (Santo 2015).

Other pharmaceutical and biotech companies will consider this dubious reward for Dendreon's pioneering innovation when their scientists discover new, breakthrough drugs. The FDA seems to be most uncomfortable approving drugs with truly novel ways of fighting diseases such as cancer. Who wants to be an innovator when the reward for taking a unique, lifesaving drug to market is financial ruin?

Chapter 27

Loss of Innovation Means Shorter Lives

We've lost at least half of our pharmaceutical innovations solely for economic reasons during clinical testing. We may have lost 80% according to the estimates reported in the first decade or so after passage of the Amendments (Chapter 24). As costs—in time and money—to take a drug from the lab bench to the marketplace have increased in the subsequent decades, we may have lost even more. I wouldn't be surprised to find that we have less than 10% of the innovations that would otherwise have been ours.

What are the costs—in money and in lives—when at least 50% of our innovative new drugs never make it to the marketplace? The answer depends on how effective the lost innovations would have been compared to the drugs that actually were approved.

Lichtenberg (2003b, 43–59) estimated that each new NCE approved between 1960 and 1997 saved about 1,200,000 life-years throughout its marketed life. Saving people from death by cardiovascular disease or stroke, which were the diseases most affected by pharmaceutical innovation during this time period, gave each patient an average increased life span of 11 years.[21]

As we've seen in Chapter 23, the number of drugs that are eventually approved is about equal to those that fail during clinical trials for economic reasons. In other words, for every new drug approved after passage of the Amendments, another innovation was lost during clinical trials because manufacturers felt that they couldn't recover their development costs. Therefore, the most-conservative estimate of lost innovations is equal to the same number of drugs (979) that were approved between 1963 and 2009.

If the lost innovations were just as effective in saving lives as those that were approved, about 106,800 million people (109,090 x 979) died prematurely. Although some lost drugs might have been more effective than ones approved, a more conservative approach would be to assume that the abandoned drugs were only 25% as effective. In that case, the abandoned drugs would have resulted in a loss of 26.7 million lives (0.25 x 106,800 million).

An estimated 100 million people died between 1963 and 2009, 88 million of them from disease. If we add to the conservative estimate of 26.7 million lives lost because of abandoned drugs, the 15.0 million lost because of Amendment-driven delays, and the 1.7 million who died because of the Amendment-driven delay in educating the public about aspirin's protective effects, then about 43.4 million people—or about 49% of those who died from disease between 1963 and 2009—each lost almost 11 years of life as a result of the Amendments. Had the loss of life been evenly distributed among the population, the average person who died after passage of the Amendments would have died 5 years prematurely.

Even though such estimates are certainly shocking, they are likely to underestimate the loss of life caused by the Amendments. For example, while we've lost at least half of innovations that are abandoned in late development because they won't be profitable (DiMasi 2001b), we've also lost those drugs, such as prostaglandins for liver disease, that never enter development primarily for economic reasons. Drugs that never enter development for economic reasons weren't included in the earlier calculation. In addition, we've conservatively estimated that the lost innovations would be only 25% as effective as today's drugs; they might have saved just as many lives as—or more than—the currently approved ones.

Finally, we have yet to estimate the loss of life caused by the shift from prevention to treatment, which resulted from the Amendments (Chapters 32–39). As we'll see, the Amendments have probably shortened the lives of almost every American. Moreover, as the side effects have rippled outward into the world, people in other countries have been affected as well.

... the present system for discovering, developing, and regulating new drugs is, by its burgeoning weight, inexorably crushing innovation to death.
—William M. Wardell, co-founder of the Tufts Center for the
Study of Drug Development, 1979

Chapter 28

Loss of Pharmaceutical Innovation Means Higher Health Care Costs

To add insult to injury, we pay for the Amendments, not only with our lives, but also with our hard-earned money as the prices for pharmaceuticals rise. When drugs to treat us are unavailable because the Amendments caused a loss of innovation, we are left with options that are even more expensive than the drugs are, even with their prices inflated by the Amendments.

For example, in the early 1990s, when cimetidine was the treatment of choice for stomach ulcers, the drug cost about $900 a year. Patients often needed 2 years of treatment. However, that drug therapy replaced a $25,000 surgery and all of the lost work and leisure time that would have accompanied it (Boston Consulting Group 1993).

Similarly, when the expensive anti-AIDS drugs approved in 1996 and later were saving patients about $2,000 per year by 1998 because they needed fewer doctor visits and other medical treatments, AIDS was no longer a death sentence (Bozzette, Joyce, McCaffrey, et al. 2001, 817–23).

Herbal and other alternatives to drugs have been used to treat ulcers and AIDS. However, most physicians are not aware of them, because of the Amendments (Chapters 32–33).

Just as we calculated the potential loss of life caused by delays and loss of innovations, we can also calculate the financial loss. For each dollar we spend on a new drug, we save about $3.65 on other types of health care costs such as hospitalization. Because we usually have to go to our doctor for a prescription, this gain is offset by $1.54 in other health care costs, such as doctor visits, for a net saving of $2.11 for each additional dollar spent on new drugs (Lichtenberg 1996, 384–88; Lichtenberg 2003b). When pharmaceutical treatments allow us to continue working (or playing) instead of staying in bed while recovering from surgery, we save an additional $1.11 that we would have otherwise lost. In other words, for every extra dollar spent on drugs, we gain about $3.22 in benefits.

When we lose pharmaceutical innovations, our only choice is to pay for medical care, which costs us about three times as much as the drugs would have. Some studies suggest that the average NCE saves six to eight times more in other medical expenditures, primarily hospitalization, than the drug costs (Lichtenberg 2007, 485–90; Lichtenberg 2002). Whatever the actual number is, most pharmaceuticals are a more economical choice than are other forms of health care.

Some critics of the drug industry complain about the high cost of pharmaceuticals without recognizing that they are more cost-effective— even with the high prices caused by the Amendments—than are other types of medical care. We could slash health care costs significantly by spending more—not less—on pharmaceutical treatments.

When a disease is already treated primarily by drugs, newer drugs save more money than old ones do, even factoring in their increased cost. Newer drugs may be just a tiny bit better than the older ones, but that can mean a big difference in overall effectiveness. For example, if a newer drug needs to be taken only once a day instead of twice a day, patients are less likely to miss a dose. Better compliance means better blood pressure or glucose control, for example, which translates into fewer hospital and doctor visits.

For every extra dollar spent on newer drugs by the general population, rather than drugs that were introduced 10 years previously, about seven times that amount is saved in other costs, primarily hospitalization. Medicare saves six times the extra costs for new drugs for the elderly, mostly from decreased hospitalization (Lichtenberg 2007). Consequently, when health insurance doesn't cover the newest drugs, patients are worse off health-wise, and the insurer pays more for other types of medical care.

Thus, government actions that discourage creation and distribution of drugs will "save" money only at enormous cost. People will die sooner. Their lives will be more painful. And other health care expenditures will rise.
—Doug Bandow, Senior Fellow at the Cato Institute

When life expectancy is extended by drugs, medical care, or preventative medicine, the economic gains are enormous. People who live longer with less disability create more wealth. Older individuals have a lifetime of education and experience to bring to bear and are generally more efficient producers than are the very young.

The increase in life expectancy between 1970 and 1998 added about $2.6 trillion (in 1996 dollars) to the wealth of the United States. Because the GDP (gross domestic product), a measure of wealth creation, was about $5.5 trillion during the same period, better health was responsible for almost half of that figure (Murphy & Topel 2003, 41–73, esp. 42).

Conversely, when at least half of our population dies prematurely because lifesaving pharmaceutical innovations are abandoned, delayed, or underused, everyone's standard of living is compromised. Living in a nation made wealthier by better health means that the average person will live longer, be paid more, have more goods and services to choose from, and be better able to afford them.

Chapter 29

The Amendments Stifled Innovation by Physicians
Stem Cell Research

I n Chapter 3, we learned how medical practice with antibiotics was altered shortly after passage of the Amendments. Combination antibiotics went from being prescribed widely to becoming grounds for potential malpractice. The FDA continues to encroach on the practice of medicine by altering the definition of what constitutes a drug.

Few people are aware of how fast our knowledge about stem cells is moving forward. Much of this research is started in the United States but has been slowed or stopped by the FDA as it extends its reach into what many regard as the practice of medicine, courtesy of the Amendments.

In March 2003, 16-year-old Dimitri Bonnville was rushed to the hospital after being shot in the heart with a nail gun. He suffered a massive heart attack; his only hope was a heart transplant or an experimental stem cell procedure. Bonnville was transferred to Beaumont Hospital in Royal Oak, Michigan, where Dr. William O'Neill and his team treated the teenager with drugs to stimulate his body's production of stem cells. Stem cells, which will take on the characteristics of the organ in which they are placed, were removed from Bonnville's blood, concentrated, and injected into his heart. Bonnville left the hospital a week later and was playing basketball just 4 months after the procedure (Epstein 2013).

Because of those exciting results, O'Neill had planned to run a clinical trial on 400 patients who had recent major heart attacks, giving stem cells to half of the patients and placebo to the other half. However, the FDA claimed that those infusions were drugs and therefore had to go through its regulatory process. The agency then deemed O'Neill's treatment to be too risky, even though one-third of the eligible patients would die without treatment over the next year (Epstein 2013). The agency wanted more animal studies before allowing the procedure in humans. The hospital wasn't equipped for animal studies, so the FDA effectively put an end to this lifesaving procedure at Beaumont.

A promising new treatment for heart attack victims was sidelined. Because heart disease is the number one killer in the United States and in most developed countries, the FDA's decision probably condemned thousands, if not tens of thousands, of people with heart problems to a premature death.

Stem cell research for heart attack victims continues in both Europe and the United States, but drug companies must use the step-by-step process demanded by regulatory agencies. By the time one of those "drugs" is approved, millions of heart attack victims who might have been saved by stem cell technology as early as 2003 will have died.

Instead of stimulating the body with drugs to make more adult stem cells, doctors can now remove them from a person's bone marrow or blood; culture them for several days to make more; and inject them back into the patient's knees, hips, or other joints. The stem cells repair the damaged tissue, often making surgery unnecessary.

Dr. Christopher Centeno in Colorado pioneered some of the techniques. The FDA didn't object when he took cells from patients and injected them into their joints the same day. However, when he multiplied them in culture so that more cells could be injected, the FDA designated those "manipulated" cells as new drugs that had to go through the costly and lengthy approval process.

Centeno moved his cultured stem cells offshore; thus, only same-day procedures remained in the United States. Patients wanting the high concentrations of stem cells made possible by culturing now must go to the Cayman Islands. Clearly, only the well-to-do can afford the more-effective procedures.

In 2010, the FDA filed a suit against Centeno's Regenerative Sciences in the hopes of getting a court to uphold its decision. In February 2014, the District of Columbia Circuit of the US Court of Appeals agreed that cultured cells were drugs under the FDA's jurisdiction (US Court of Appeals 2014). This decision has discouraged a great deal of stem cell research that would have otherwise improved—and even saved—our lives. Each cultured stem cell product will have to go through the expensive FDA approval process designed for new drugs.

Consequently, when doctors try to work with the FDA in stem cell research, the process is much slower than it otherwise should be. By 2014, the FDA had approved only five stem cell products, all of which are for diseases of the blood and immune system (Rosemann 2014, 2073–76).

Even when results with stem cells show unprecedented promise, the long FDA-mandated development pathway causes frustration. For example, when Ted Harada was diagnosed with ALS (amyotrophic lateral sclerosis), or Lou Gehrig's disease, in 2010, he was told that there was no cure. He rapidly deteriorated to the point where he couldn't walk to his mailbox or even open a zippered storage bag.

However, Ted had the good fortune to enroll in a clinical trial at Emory University, just 45 minutes from his home near Atlanta. The procedure had never been done before: surgeons would open up the spinal cord and inject fetal stem cells directly into it, bypassing the blood-brain barrier.

Unexpectedly, Ted made unprecedented progress, becoming the first person *ever* to see a reversal of ALS symptoms. After 10 months, he began to weaken again, so the doctors repeated the procedure in August 2012. Just 2 months later, he made a 2.5-mile walk for ALS.

Ted was fortunate; the FDA had allowed treatment with only about a tenth of the stem cell dose that the doctors had originally wanted to use. However, if Ted's symptoms return, he won't be allowed another dose, because he will no longer meet the eligibility criteria for the clinical trial (Olsen 2015, 1–18).

About 40 patients have been treated in the clinical trials so far; about 50% responded with improvement or slowing of the disease. Not surprisingly, the best responders are the ones who had lost the least amount of function when they received the treatment (Neuralstem Inc. 2016; N566 2016).

About 5,600 patients are diagnosed annually with ALS; at any one time, about 30,000 people in the United States are living with the disease. However, it will be several years before this procedure gains FDA approval—if it ever does. Neuralstem, the company that is taking this stem cell "drug" through the clinical development process, was still in Phase 2 trials at the end of 2017 (Neuralstem Pipeline n.d.).

In the meantime, ALS patients have little or no hope of effective treatment. Instead, like the AIDS patients, they are desperately seeking to acquire drugs now in clinical trials, even if they have to make the drugs in their own kitchen laboratories (Marcus 2012). If the courts had ruled that stem cell infusions were medical treatments, instead of drugs, people with ALS might already have a better alternative.

More than 100,000 women each year opt for breast reconstruction after surgical mastectomies for cancer (American Society of Plastic Surgeons 2016). Stem cell breast reconstruction was popularized by a well-known actress, Suzanne Somers, who had her procedure videotaped (Somers 2011). Instead of a massive "tummy tuck" to obtain fat for the reconstruction, her doctor took only a syringe full of abdominal fat to harvest her stem cells.

Unfortunately for American women, the FDA has decided that because breasts are meant to produce milk, using abdominal fat to harvest stem cells makes them nonhomologous (US FDA 2014; Jaffe 2016). Simply stated, the FDA believes that if stem cells from one part of the body are used to alter another, *different*, part, then the stem cells are drugs and are subject to its extensive regulatory process. Should the FDA continue to maintain this position, women who want this less-invasive reconstruction will have to go offshore. Only women who can afford such travel will have access to it.

Typical breast reconstruction after mastectomy uses abdominal fat rather than only the stem cells that can be isolated from it. Will the FDA decide that using abdominal fat is also nonhomologous and ban it too?

Chapter 30

The Amendments Stifled Innovation by Physicians
Cancer Treatments

E ven before the passage of the Amendments, the FDA seemed to have a bias against therapies originated by practicing physicians. The FDA and state medical boards often collaborated in prosecuting doctors working toward cancer cures, such as Harry Hoxey (Hoxey Herbal Therapy); Andrew C. Ivey (Krebiozen); William Frederick Koch (synthetic antitoxins, glyoxilide, and benzoquinone); and Robert E. Lincoln (the cancer-killing bacteriophage, *Staphage lifsate*) (Ausubel 2000, 118–34).

Rather than encourage testing of those supposed cures, the regulators sought to criminalize, jail, or revoke the medical licenses of the physicians. The attitude toward innovators appears to be "guilty of quackery until proven innocent."

Despite the government's (FDA) multimillion dollar prosecution which included falsified testimony, later confessed by the government, the four defendants (including Dr. Stephen Druovic and Dr. Andrew Ivy) were acquitted.... [Moreover,] the jury went to extraordinary lengths to say it believed Krebiozen had merit and should be tested, based on the positive, well-documented testimony it had heard.
—David Rorvik, "A Defense of Unorthodoxy," *Harper's Magazine*, June 1976

In 7 years after passage of the Amendment, the FDA stopped more than 250 ongoing clinical investigations of new drugs (Wardell & Lasagna 1975, 22). More than 80% of those clinical trials were being done by single investigators, usually doctors, because the FDA felt that not enough animal work had been done (Jadlow 1970, 158). Before the Amendments, each individual investigator or physician decided how much animal work should be done before testing in humans. In 1982, FDA Bureau of Drugs Director Richard Crout articulated the FDA's bias against physicians, stating, "I never have and never will approve a new drug to an individual, but only to a large pharmaceutical firm with unlimited finances" (Spotlight 1982).

The expense of drug development is now so large that even an affluent individual would have a difficult time funding it. An FDA examiner who approved a drug that didn't have a truckload of studies backing it would be open to censure should its side effects, which every drug has, come to congressional attention.

This attitude may explain, in part, the FDA's continued assault on Dr. Stanislaw Burzynski and his antineoplastons for cancer. I first heard of Burzynski in the early 1980s, when he was treating an associate of mine. This gentleman had already outlived the death sentence given to him by his oncologists. Like many of Burzynski's patients, he attributed his longevity to the antineoplastons with which Burzynski treated him. However, after gaining an additional decade of good health, the cancer finally killed him.

Burzynski (1976, 275–79) discovered small proteins in the blood and urine of healthy adults that were absent in cancer patients. He believed that those antineoplastons turned on and off the genes that controlled cancer growth. He isolated the proteins and eventually made them in his laboratory for his Texas patients. Because the FDA regulations apply only to drugs sold through interstate commerce, Burzynski's attorneys advised him that he was legally able to do so (Burzynski 1977).

Cancer patients who had not responded to other treatments began coming to Burzynski as their last hope. Some of them survived and credited the antineoplaston treatment.

In 1983, the FDA asked the courts to close Burzynski's clinic on the grounds that he was violating their regulations. US District Court Judge Gabrielle McDonald for the Southern District of Texas disagreed with the FDA and ruled that as long as Burzynski confined his activities to the state of Texas, he could continue his work (Life Extension Foundation 2010, 474).

In 1985, the FDA conducted a raid of Burzynski's clinic, seizing 200,000 documents. Medical records of his patients were taken, putting those patients at risk as a result of loss of their histories and test results. To recover the medical records, Burzynski had to install a copier at the FDA, send someone to make copies, and return the copies to the clinic— all at the doctor's own expense (Life Extension Foundation 2010, 475).

In spite of the "evidence" obtained on this raid, the federal grand jury still refused to indict Burzynski. In 1986, the FDA conducted another raid and once again failed to gain an indictment.

Burzynski believes that the Texas Medical Board has been collaborating with the FDA against him. In 1990, the Texas Medical Board filed a complaint that FDA regulations were not being followed and threatened to revoke his license to practice medicine. Judge Earl Corbitt ruled in favor of Burzynski because the Texas Medical Board had produced no evidence that Burzynski was harming patients. Furthermore, the FDA regulations did not apply unless interstate commerce was involved (Texas Medical Board n.d.).

In March 1995, after Burzynski appeared on *CBS This Morning*, the FDA conducted still another raid. This raid was especially puzzling, because the Office of Alternative Medicine (OAM) had been working with Burzynski to evaluate antineoplastons under INDs approved by the FDA. Less than a week before the raid, Dr. Freddie Ann Hoffman of the FDA met with representatives from the OAM and had a positive discussion about some of those collaborations.

In July 1995, Congress held a hearing on the FDA's baffling actions against Burzynski. Congress was concerned that the FDA was abusing its power. Shortly after the hearings closed, Burzynski was indicted on

November 20, 1995, and charged with 75 counts of fraud and federal law violations. Burzynski (1995) faced a maximum of 290 years in a federal prison, as well as $18.5 million dollars in fines.

Federal prosecutors concede that a cancer doctor they will put on trial here in January for using an innovative but unapproved drug has been "saving lives." The admission is a landmark in the Food and Drug Administration's 13-year campaign against Dr. Stanislaw Burzynski, whose patients have raised more than $700,000 for his legal defense.
—Thomas D. Elias, "Doctor's Lifesaving Effort Could Land Him in Prison: FDA Ignores Cancer Drug's Success," *Washington Times*, December 5, 1996

Judge Simeon Lake of the US District Court for the Southern District of Texas ruled that Burzynski had to administer the antineoplastons exclusively through FDA-approved clinical trials as a condition of his "continued pretrial release" (Quickwatch 1998). Working with the FDA, Burzynski set up more than 70 INDs, which would allow him to treat his present and future cancer patients. Once the FDA had oversight of Burzynski's anti-neoplaston treatment, their case was severely compromised. After all, Burzynski had made a good faith effort at cooperation; the FDA had approved his INDs. Jurors could not understand why they were being asked to send him to prison. By May 27, 1997, Burzynski had prevailed on all charges (Life Extension Foundation 2010).

That was not the end of the story, however. In 2012, 6-year-old Josia Cotto died from complications of the antineoplaston treatment (Orac 2013). The FDA put a partial hold on Burzynski's studies but later lifted it because he was working with the FDA on a protocol for Phase 3 studies (Szabo 2014). However, Phase 3 studies are notoriously expensive. Burzynski is unlikely to afford them with his mounting legal bills. Instead, he will likely have to bill patients, so only the affluent will be able to afford his treatment.

In 2015, the Texas Medical Board sued Burzynski for allegedly harming patients through unethical practices in his clinic and, at that time, intended to revoke his license to practice medicine (Texas State Office 2015). The court issued a Proposal for Decision for the Texas Medical Board to review before deciding whether or not to proceed with the suit. Although the proposal indicated that Burzynski should have (a) provided patients with more explanation of their medical bills, (b) disclosed his financial interest in the pharmacy supplying their medicines, and (c) done a better job of giving them informed consent, the Proposal concludes with, "If Respondent [Burzynski] is unable to continue practicing medicine, critically ill cancer patients being treated with ANP [atrial natriuretic peptide] under FDA-approved clinical trials or a special exception will no longer have access to this treatment. Respondent's continued practice in treating advanced cancer patients is a present value to the cancer community. Respondent's treatments have saved the lives of cancer patients, both adults and children, who were not expected to live."

Clearly, Judge Lesli G. Ginn believes that Burzynski's license should not be revoked (Texas Medical Board 2016). Ultimately, the Texas Medical Board opted to put the doctor on probation and fine him $60,000, which Burzynski's attorneys considered a win (Chang 2017).

Clearly, Burzynski believes wholeheartedly in his antineoplastons. Would anyone but a true believer continue to treat patients through decades of scorn, litigation, and crippling legal bills?

Obviously, many of his patients do too because 60 of them signed a petition to the Texas Medical Board asking it to stop harassing the doctor. Some researchers, who have evaluated his cases or treated their own patients with Burnzynksi's neoplastons, are enthusiastic as well (Burdick 1997; Ogata, Matono, Tsuda, et al. 2015; Patronas 1993).

If we attempt to imprison doctors who have innovative ideas about deadly diseases, how many innovations might we lose? How many researchers with less grit than Burzynski have forsaken a potential cancer cure for fear of ridicule and legal sanctions? If our regulatory system sues, rather than encourages, doctors who have new ideas about disease, how many of them will dare to innovate?

While heart disease has plummeted during the past half-century, cancer patients have not fared as well over the same period. Most increases in cancer survival are due to early detection, not to advances in treatment. Perhaps prosecution of innovators, made possible by the Amendments, is part of the reason.

Chapter 31

The Costs of the
Amendments Are Not
Offset by Their Benefits

I f the Amendments gave us safer, more effective drugs, we might be willing to pay the additional costs that they imposed, both in higher drug prices and fewer innovations. After all, taking ineffective drugs off the market might offset the increasing amounts we pay at the pharmacy. If the Amendments kept unsafe drugs off the market, fewer people would die. How do the costs of the Amendments compare to the savings that they give us?

DID THE AMENDMENTS GIVE US MORE EFFECTIVE DRUGS?

The Amendments were supposed to ensure that only effective drugs reached the marketplace to protect the consumer from wasteful spending. As mentioned earlier (Chapter 3), the FDA asked the National Academy of Sciences to evaluate the drugs already on the market.

The FDA had instructed the panels to rate drugs as "ineffective," "possibly effective," "probably effective," or "effective" for each "indication" (medical problem) for which they were sold (NRC 1969, 7). The National Academy rated about 7% of prescription drugs, most of which were once "new chemical entities," or NCEs, as lacking substantial evidence of effectiveness for any of the indications for which they were sold (NRC 1969, 12). The FDA pulled those drugs from the market. In an independent evaluation of the National Academy data, Dr. James Jondrow (1972) at the University of Wisconsin concluded that evidence of effectiveness was lacking for as many as 9% of pre-Amendment prescription drugs.

Peltzman compared the types of drugs carried by both pharmacies and hospital formularies. He found that the groups did not, as might be expected, order only drugs approved after passage of the Amendments and shun ones marketed before 1962. Indeed, he could find no difference in the ordering behavior of formularies and pharmacies in regards to whether or not a drug had been marketed pre- or post-Amendment.

He did find that the American Medical Association rated drugs approved post-Amendment to be slightly more effective. Prescribing physicians believed about 10% of the drugs approved after 1962 were ineffective, as opposed to 20% for drugs approved before that date. In other words, physicians believed that consumers might expect to save as much as 10% of their total pharmacy bill because of the Amendments (Peltzman 1974).

Clearly, the marketplace had already eliminated most, but not all, of the ineffective drugs. Physicians who often prescribed a drug were usually able to tell if a drug worked for their patients. If a drug wasn't effective, doctors would stop prescribing it, and pharmaceutical companies would stop making it.

Even if a drug was effective for one indication, it didn't always work for others, even though it was marketed for those extra indications before 1962. However, because doctors were able to tell about 90% of the time if a drug worked, it's unlikely that consumers wasted much money on drugs that worked for one indication but not another.

Of course, even the best drugs aren't effective for everyone who uses them. Like it or not, as consumers we will sometimes buy drugs that don't work for us. Our science is not currently good enough to save us from that "waste"; we don't know how to make drugs that work for every person. Different genetics, environmental stresses, and undiagnosed inefficiencies in our body's biochemistry can positively or negatively impact each drug's effectiveness in ways we don't completely understand. The average drug works in about half of the people it's intended to treat (Conner 2003). To muddy the waters further, even "ineffective" drugs can cure people through the placebo effect. Consequently, one might argue that there is no such thing as an ineffective drug.

The Amendments may have saved us from the 10% of ineffective drugs that were on the market, but at what cost? Clearly, today's drugs have been made much more expensive—perhaps as much as 40 times what they otherwise would have been (Chapter 19)—because of the tripling of development time and exponential increases in the costs of studies necessary for approval. The effectiveness studies are one of the most-expensive regulatory requirements and cost consumers many times more than the waste that they supposedly prevent.

Consumers might be willing to pay higher prices for drugs if the Amendments gave them more safety. After all, safer drugs mean less loss of life through deadly side effects. Like effectiveness, safety is sometimes difficult to define. For example, we tolerate serious side effects with cancer drugs that we wouldn't accept in a headache remedy. Therefore, to determine whether the Kefauver-Harris Amendments have delivered on their promise of safer drugs, we will look at several indicators.

DID THE AMENDMENTS GIVE US SAFER DRUGS?

When drugs are approved by the FDA and subsequently found to be unsafe, they are withdrawn from the market. If the Amendments actually protected us from unsafe drugs, the withdrawal rate after the Amendments should be less than before their passage. Indeed, this was the Amendments' implied promise to the American people: fewer unsafe drugs would reach the market.

The Prescription Drug User Fee Act (PDUFA), which will be discussed in detail later in this chapter, was passed in October 1992. In brief, this act allowed drug companies to pay a "user fee" that would be used to hire more FDA examiners to speed the approval process. An unusually high number of withdrawals occurred in the years immediately after PDUFA, creating concern that the shortened review time was allowing unsafe drugs to get to the market (Olson 2002, 615–31; Olson 2008, 175–200).

However, this trend did not continue. Later studies indicated that withdrawal rates did not differ for drugs approved in the decades immediately before and after PDUFA (Berndt, Gottschalk, Philipson, et al. 2005, 547–51). The withdrawal rate was 3.4% from 1962 to 1992 and 3.3% from 1993 to 2011, confirming that PDUFA had no influence on this parameter (Bakke, Manocchia, de Abajo, et al. 1995, 108–17; US FDA 2005a, 42, 43; Wikipedia. n.d.; Throckmorton 2014, 6).

How do those withdrawal rates compare to pre-Amendment ones? Of the drugs approved between 1947 and 1961, the withdrawal rate was 2.5% because of safety concerns (Gieringer 1985; Wikipedia n.d.; Bakke, Wardell, & Lasagna 1984, 559–67). Clearly, withdrawal rates did not go down after the Amendments. They might not have gone up significantly either, because the difference between pre- and post-Amendment withdrawal rates is small.

Finding no difference between pre- and post-Amendment withdrawal rates is exactly what we would expect to see if lack of knowledge, rather than manufacturer negligence in testing, was responsible for most withdrawals. The Amendments did not deliver on their promise that fewer dangerous drugs would make it to the US market.

DID COUNTRIES WITH LESS REGULATION HAVE GREATER WITHDRAWAL RATES?

Another way to look at the negative impact of the Amendments on safety is to examine the withdrawal rates in countries with less-stringent regulations. Although Britain did add some safety regulations in the mid-1960s and some effectiveness requirements in the early 1970s, they were considerably less demanding than those in the United States. Consequently, as described in Chapter 9, new drugs reached the British market earlier. Fewer innovations were lost. Consequently, the United Kingdom had an average of 21 new drugs each year in the 1970s, while the United States had only 16 (Bakke, Wardell, & Lasagna 1984).

Had the Amendments protected the United States from unsafe drugs, Britain's withdrawal rate would have been higher than that of the United States. If scientific ignorance, rather than lack of regulation, was responsible for most of the withdrawals, the two countries would be comparable. The United Kingdom had a slightly higher withdrawal rate than did the United States (4% vs. 3%) for drugs approved between 1974 and 1993. However, the difference was unlikely to be significant because Spain, with even less-stringent drug regulation than both of the two other countries, had a 3% withdrawal rate, just as the United States did (Bakke, Manocchia, de Abajo, et al. 1995).

Because more drugs were approved in the United Kingdom, more were withdrawn, even though the *percentage* in both countries was similar. Britain would have experienced more side effects overall than the United States did. However, the British would also have quicker access to more lifesaving drugs. Which country benefited more?

Dr. Dale Gieringer of Stanford University estimated that, without the Amendments, 5,000–10,000 US lives would have been lost had the FDA approved the same drugs that Britain had. However, Americans would have gotten lifesaving drugs earlier without the Amendments, saving about 21,000–120,000 lives (Gieringer 1985, 196). In other words, Gieringer found that delays in approvals were more deadly than the extra side effects that came from a more rapid approval process.

Using different methodology, Dr. Sam Peltzman calculated a 4:1 cost-to-benefit ratio for the 1962 Amendments in 1974 (Peltzman 1974). According to those two studies, the Amendments appeared to be—quite literally—regulatory overkill.

HOW MANY LIVES DID THE AMENDMENTS SAVE?

Even early studies found that the Amendments did more harm than good, probably because most of the safety problems that existed before their passage were due to scientific ignorance, rather than to manufacturer neglect. The frequency of severe side effects in the 1960s and 1970s was low relative to the lifesaving benefits of new pharmaceuticals.

Dr. Dale Gieringer (1985), for example, reviewed published data about the drugs that had killed or seriously harmed more than 100 people in the United States between 1950 and 1962. Table 2 lists those drugs and the estimated number of deaths and serious casualties. Gieringer included the Cutter vaccine in his analysis, so it is listed in Table 2 for the sake of completeness, even though the NCE and NME numbers cited in this book elsewhere do not include vaccines.

Chloramphenicol, which caused an estimated 753 deaths over a 6-year period (Peltzman 1974, 53–54), was a powerful antibiotic that had a rare and usually fatal side effect, aplastic anemia, which occurred in 1 out of every 25,000–50,000 patients (Gieringer 1985). Even today, antibiotics are tested on a few thousand people before marketing, so this side effect could still have been missed had chloramphenicol been approved post-Amendment.

Table 2. The Number of Americans Experiencing Serious Side Effects with Drugs Approved 1950–62.[22]

Drug	Deaths	Serious Casualties
Chloramphencicol	753	
MER-29		400–500
Cutter vaccine	11	204
Orabilex	25–100	
Total	864	704

Even after this fatal side effect was widely publicized, however, physicians continued to prescribe chloramphenicol because of its effectiveness, especially against some hard-to-kill microbes (Peltzman 1974, 53–54). In spite of a life-threatening side effect in small numbers of patients, chloramphenicol could save enough lives that both the FDA and the medical profession felt it was the antibiotic of choice in certain types of deadly infections. It remains on the market today, even though it killed more Americans than any other drug in the 12 years before passage of the Amendments.

MER-29, a cholesterol-lowering NCE approved in 1960, was withdrawn a couple of years later, because it was found to cause cataracts after prolonged use (Laughlin & Carey 1962, 339–40; Kirby 1962, 543–44). Richardson-Merrell, the company making the drug, had seen cataracts in their dog studies but thought (erroneously) that they were reversible (Sallmann, Grimes, & Collins 1963, 49–60, esp. 59). Because the Amendments required all animal data on each drug to be submitted to the FDA along with the request for approval, this type of side effect would probably have been caught if the Amendments had been in effect.

Richardson-Merrell was the company trying to bring thalidomide into the United States. Had the FDA approved thalidomide, the company's reputation would have been badly battered by introducing two dangerous drugs within a couple years of each other. Branding was much more important in the years before the Amendments, because physicians often looked at a company's reputation for quality when deciding whether to be one of the first to give their patients a new drug. Upjohn's founder, W. E. Upjohn, for example, coined the company's motto "Keep the quality up!" in the 1880s to inspire trusted products.

Today, much less consideration is given to the maker of the new drug. When the Amendments empowered the FDA, the agency's approval became the primary consideration of quality, creating less incentive for pharmaceutical firms to protect their reputation.

Cutter Laboratories was one of several facilities that produced the Salk polio vaccine. In 1955, Cutter distributed a batch in which the live virus had not been fully inactivated, resulting in a couple hundred cases of polio and close to a dozen deaths. The problem wasn't unique to Cutter: other producers also had trouble inactivating the virus (Offit 2005, 100, 116–19, 133). The NIH Laboratory of Biologics Control had evidently ignored the results of its own testing and certified the vaccine anyway (Shorter 1987, 68–70). The Amendments probably wouldn't have prevented this tragedy, because the government agency, not the company, was found negligent (Offit 2005). Although the Cutter vaccine was not considered an NCE, it is included for completeness from Gieringer's research.

To put the pre-Amendment drug side effects in perspective, had thalidomide been approved in the United States, we might have expected between 10,000 and 19,000 children to be affected (Gieringer 1985, 193). However, regulations in place at the time were clearly sufficient to prevent its approval. The Amendments were not needed.

Thalidomide was the most-devastating drug tragedy of its time, causing more deaths and serious injuries than all other dangerous drugs marketed in the decades before the Amendments combined. The months between taking thalidomide and the birth of a deformed infant delayed the discovery of thalidomide's negative impact on the unborn baby, greatly increasing the number of children affected.

Thalidomide-type products do not appear to have been introduced frequently in the years before 1962.

—Dr. Sam Peltzman, American Enterprise Institute and University of Chicago

If we make the optimistic—and surely the unrealistic—assumption that the Amendments could have prevented a thalidomide-like tragedy every 12 years, as well as *all* of the side effects listed in Table 2, how many lives might they have saved? Using the maximum number of deaths plus casualties from Table 2 (1,568) and adding in the maximum number of 19,000 US children who would have been affected had thalidomide been approved (20,568), we estimate the maximum number of lives that could potentially have been saved by the Amendments: 17,140 per decade.

In the 50 years between 1963 and 2012, a maximum of 85,700 people might have been saved from death or serious harm. Because the population increased during this time, the number of casualties would have too. After making an adjustment for population growth, perhaps as many as 128,283 people might have been saved by the Amendments through 2012, making the unrealistic assumption that we would have had a thalidomide-like tragedy every 15 years and that *every* drug side effect that killed or maimed more than 100 people before 1962 would have been eliminated by the Amendments.

Comparing our conservative estimate of the number of people killed by the Amendments (43.4 million; see Chapter 27) to the number that could have possibly been saved by the Amendments—at most about 128,283 individuals—the Amendments caused the premature deaths of at least 338 people for each one that they might have saved. If we estimate the negative impact of the Amendments with less-conservative assumptions, the number of people killed by the Amendments per person saved could easily quadruple.

Even if some of the estimates used to make those calculations are off by a factor of 100, the conclusion—that the Amendments' side effects outweigh their benefits—will not change. In addition, other deadly aspects of the Amendments have not yet been considered. In the next section, we'll explore reasons the post-Amendment drugs might actually have more side effects—regardless of withdrawal rate—than pre-Amendment ones had.

ARE POST-AMENDMENT DRUGS MORE DANGEROUS THAN PRE-AMENDMENT ONES?

From a scientific viewpoint, it's easy to see how the Amendments may have made today's drugs less safe. The Amendments discourage manufacturers from promoting older drugs with known side effects so those drugs can treat a disease different from the one for which the drugs were initially approved, because the FDA takes as long to approve a second "indication" as it did to approve the first (DiMasi, Brown, & Lasagna 1996, 315–37).

In addition, if the patent is close to expiration, it might not make financial sense to undertake the extra studies that the FDA demands, especially if those costs can't be made up before the drug undergoes generic competition. Instead, in hopes of having a chance at recovering the development costs, a manufacturer may choose to restart the development process with a new drug that has many more years of patent protection.

Because no amount of testing will predict every side effect, the American public is exposed to additional risks with every new drug. With older drugs, the risk profile is better known and is less likely to produce unwanted safety surprises.

In addition, the large and ever-increasing costs of taking a drug from the lab bench to the market has shifted the focus of development from short-term to long-term treatments to increase the chances that the manufacturer can recover costs. Our bodies have many ways to detoxify drugs, but taking those drugs every day for years, or even decades, can overwhelm our livers or kidneys, as well as deplete essential nutrients in the process. Eventually, the loss of nutrients or other stresses of detoxification create problems that can be life-threatening.

The number of marketed drugs has increased every year, even though some drugs become obsolete and are no longer sold. As older people exhibit more symptoms of declining health, doctors have more drugs available to treat them with, so prescriptions per patient naturally increase. The dangerous downside of this approach, however, is the almost certain increase in interactions between drugs, which can create deadly side effects of their own.

Indeed, when researchers combined a number of studies, they estimated deaths from *properly* prescribed drugs in 1994 alone to be about 106,000 (Lazarou, Pomeranz, & Corey 1998, 1200–05), suggesting that prescription drugs are the fourth to sixth leading cause of death in the United States. Critics of this study point out that a considerable amount of guesswork went into the evaluations (Kvasz, Allen, Gordon, et al. 2000). A 2011 study suggested that about 128,000–256,000 deaths might be attributable to pharmaceuticals (Institute for Safe Medication Practices 2012), only 14% of which weren't preventable by better prescribing, patient compliance, etc. (Howard, Avery, Slavenburg, & Royal 2007, 136–47). Even if only 35,840 (256,000 x 0.14) annual deaths fall into this latter category, post-Amendment pharmaceuticals would appear to be responsible for more fatalities than pre-Amendment ones ever were.

Does this finding mean that post-Amendment drugs have more side effects than pre-Amendment ones did? That's certainly a possibility, but drug–drug interactions are probably at least partially to blame. Drugs can save lives, but using too many together can backfire. A patient who tolerates a dozen medications might be placed in a life-threatening situation when a 13th drug is added. Today, doctors tend to prescribe more medications per person than in pre-Amendment days.

THE AMENDMENTS CREATE THE BIGGEST DRUG DISASTER OF ALL

The American people believed that the Amendments would keep deadly drugs from the marketplace, even though the Amendments actually focused on effectiveness, rather than safety. Unfortunately, Vioxx, the greatest drug disaster in US history, happened *after* Amendment passage.

Vioxx—approved in 1999 and withdrawn from the market in 2004—was designed to be easier on the stomach than were the other anti-inflammatory drugs used to treat arthritis. Unfortunately, it also doubled the rate of serious cardiovascular events such as heart attacks and strokes (Ross, Madigan, Hill, et al. 2009, 1976–85).

The Vioxx story illustrates three important principles of pharmaceutical development: how lack of scientific knowledge plays a role in drug side effects, how the Amendments aggravate the tendency of industrial scientists to face unpleasant facts about their products, and how political pressures can cause regulators to ignore the warning signs when evaluating new drugs.

Aspirin, as well as other anti-inflammatory drugs such as Motrin® (ibuprofen), work by altering the balance of eicosanoids in the body. When Upjohn first marketed Motrin in the United States, the company received letters from arthritis sufferers expressing gratitude for a product that alleviated so much of their pain. Motrin altered the eicosanoid balance by inhibiting COX-2, a protein that was activated during inflammation to make the prostaglandins that lead to pain.

However, like all drugs, Motrin had side effects, especially when taken on a daily basis for years, which many arthritis sufferers did. In addition to inhibiting COX-2, Motrin inhibited COX-1, stopping the formation of "cytoprotective" prostaglandins that kept the stomach from digesting itself. As a result, some chronic Motrin users developed stomach ulcers. Although most people recovered when they stopped taking Motrin, some did not. They had to be hospitalized, and some died from gastric bleeding.

Vioxx, a COX-2 inhibitor, was supposed to relieve pain without inhibiting COX-1 in the stomach. Vioxx was intended to be a safer anti-inflammatory drug.

However, prostacyclin, the eicosanoid in the blood that prevents platelets from clumping and thereby thwarts heart attacks (Chapter 15), was made not just by COX-1 but also by COX-2 as well, at least in humans (FitzGerald 2003, 879–90). Prostacyclin's dependence on COX-2 wasn't widely recognized until after Vioxx was marketed. Suppressing COX-2 caused prostacyclin in the blood to plummet (FitzGerald 2004, 1709–11), causing more platelet clumping and more heart attacks.

However, Vioxx's propensity to cause heart attacks was suspected even before the drug was approved. Because of this concern, the FDA's Advisory Committee began to evaluate the accumulating data from the Vioxx trials shortly after its approval and published their results 2 years later. Vioxx caused significantly more heart attacks compared to placebo ($p<0.04$, for the technically inclined) (Mukherjee, Nissen, & Topol 2001,

954–59). However, the only action taken by the FDA was to change the drug's package insert—a couple of years later—to include cardiovascular problems as a possible side effect (Graham 2004; Bhattacharya 2005). Why didn't the FDA remove Vioxx from the market?

Part of the problem was the Prescription Drug User Fee Act (PDFUA), passed in 1992. This act allowed pharmaceutical firms to pay the FDA "user fees" for each approval they sought. The FDA would hire new reviewers with this money so that NDAs could be reviewed more rapidly. This process shaved about a year from the drug development process (see Figure 1 for the negative impact of PDUFA on drug development times) (Kaitin & Cairns 2003). Fewer people died waiting for new drugs, which was obviously a good thing. The drug lag was partially reversed. Of the NCEs approved between 1999 and 2001, 51% were first marketed in the United States (Kaitlin & Cairns 2003, 357–71).

However, new regulations, like new drugs, often have unwanted side effects. In 1993, the user fee for the typical NCE was $100,000; by 2018, the user fee had soared to $2,421,495 (US FDA 2017a). In 2016, user fees provided 72% of the total budget for PFUDA, while congressional appropriations provided the rest (US FDA 2017b, 16). The FDA collects enough money from PFUDA that it has had to carry over funds to the next fiscal year for the past decade or so (US FDA 2017b, 9). Funding the FDA in this manner has created some ethical problems. Instead of being beholden only to Congress for their paychecks, the FDA is now beholden, in equal measure, to the firms that they are supposed to regulate.

The approval of Vioxx is a good indication of how this ethical conflict endangers the American public. Dr. David Graham of the FDA pointed out the Vioxx safety issues to his management. Graham's supervisor blatantly told him that the FDA's client was the pharmaceutical industry, not Congress or even the American public. According to Graham, the FDA now tries hard to approve a drug, even if it's only for limited uses (Loudon 2005). After all, if drug companies don't make money, they can't fund future R&D, and the FDA can't collect user fees to support its personnel. PDFUA has created a severe conflict of interest for the FDA, thereby ensuring that the American public will be exposed to more unsafe drugs in the future.

Graham and his collaborators in the FDA's Office of Drug Safety analyzed data from Kaiser Permanente in California and found that Vioxx caused up to 3.5 times as many cardiac events as did Celebrex, another COX-2 inhibitor (Graham, Campen, Hui, et al. 2005, 475–81). Graham estimated that about 140,000 heart attacks and 60,000 deaths were attributable to Vioxx (Loudon 2005). If those estimates are correct, Vioxx would probably be the greatest drug disaster of all time.

Graham's estimates are probably conservative. As many as 80 million patients may have taken Vioxx before the manufacturer voluntarily withdrew it from the market. Because some studies suggested that Vioxx caused as many as 16 excess heart attacks and strokes per 1,000 people (Topol 2004, 1707–09), as many as 1,280,000 individuals could have experienced one of those serious side effects in the 5 years Vioxx was sold.

In his testimony to Congress, Graham indicated that his superior in the Office of Drug Safety pressured him to change his conclusions about Vioxx and his talk at an upcoming International Conference on Pharmacoepidemiology in Bordeaux, France, in August 2004 (Graham, Campen, Hui, et al. 2005; Bhattacharya 2005). Graham refused. Merck withdrew Vioxx from the market a month after Graham publically shared his results.

I would argue that the FDA, as currently configured, is incapable of protecting America against another Vioxx. We are virtually defenseless.
—Dr. David Graham, FDA Office of Drug Safety

Graham claimed his superiors at the FDA threatened him with severe consequences if he published his full-length paper subsequent to the meeting (CNN 2005). When he was scheduled to testify before Congress, the Acting FDA Commissioner offered Graham a promotion, which he viewed as a bribe to remain silent (Loudon 2005).

Finding problems with a marketed drug suggests that the FDA was wrong to approve Vioxx in the first place. Sometimes it is psychologically easier to be in denial rather than admit to a mistake.

In addition, given all the unknowns in pharmacology, we simply can't always predict safety problems that will occur until a large number of people actually take a drug. The virtually constant withdrawal rate in the 50 years suggests that we can expect about 3–4% of approved drugs to be withdrawn eventually for safety reasons that can't be predicted even with all the Amendment-driven studies.

Unfortunately, no drug is perfectly safe or always effective. In spite of our best efforts, we will have some drug casualties. No regulation can keep us perfectly safe. Poorly designed regulations can have more deadly side effects than the drugs themselves can.

Many regulations are put in place with the support, the encouragement, and even the instigation of the industry being regulated. Established companies and practices are usually grandfathered in. Steep requirements are put in place for newcomers or those who are doing things differently. Competition is diminished; prices rise along with profits for the few (usually large) companies left standing through the grandfathering process (Ruwart 2015, 53–150).

When regulations become so strict that they threaten even established companies, the industry's survival depends on its ability to co-opt the regulatory process. Clearly, the long development times wrought by the Amendments created incentives for the drug companies to speed approvals through PDUFA, for the FDA to raise user fees, and for the pharmaceutical industry to influence regulators through its funding of the FDA (Ruwart 2015, 112–16).

In addition, the Amendment-driven regulatory climate fosters denial of dangerous side effects not only at the FDA, but also in the pharmaceutical companies. Scientists can spend more than a decade trying to meet the development challenges for a new drug. In a very real sense, the drug becomes their baby. When parents are told that their child has misbehaved, the first reaction is often denial. Pharmaceutical employees are human beings too. When the data suggest that their baby is a killer rather than a lifesaver, they naturally look for other explanations.

With the shorter development times before the Amendments, such psychology was still undoubtedly at play, but abandoning a drug after a year or 2 is much easier than abandoning it after 10 or 12. In addition, much more money is spent in the latter case, and the financial blow to the company is considerably greater. The more that a company has to lose, the harder it is to give up on a particular drug.

For example, in the case of Vioxx, one of the most-compelling studies compared it to naproxen, another anti-inflammatory drug. When the Vioxx group showed five times as many heart attacks as the naproxen group, Merck's explanation was that naproxen must be protecting the heart, not that Vioxx was harming it. Later studies demonstrated that just the opposite was true; once the evidence became undeniable, Merck withdrew Vioxx from the market. Graham believes that the FDA might never have withdrawn Vioxx if the manufacturer hadn't (Steinreich 2005). Indeed, Celebrex, another COX-2 inhibitor that seems to increase heart attacks—although possibly to a lesser extent—is still sold in the United States.

The loss of innovation brought about by the Amendments means that today's companies may not be able to easily replace a drug that has already undergone human testing and is found to be flawed. When I was at Upjohn, we usually had more drug candidates than we could possibly develop. However, as development costs rise and innovation decreases, companies have fewer substitutes for drugs that fail to perform as expected. Giving up on a drug that is almost at the finish line becomes even more painful.

My intent is not to excuse the denial of a drug's safety problems but rather to point out that this very real aspect of human behavior is aggravated by the regulatory climate. In both the FDA and the drug companies, the same people who supported the development and approval of a new drug are usually the ones who must decide whether or not to withdraw it. The Amendments, by creating ever-increasing development timelines and costs, make acknowledging safety problems with a new drug even more painful for both regulators and pharmaceutical executives. Perhaps that is why Vioxx made it to the market in spite of safety concerns known to both the FDA and Merck (Matthews & Martinez 2004, A1).

WOULD VIOXX HAVE STILL BEEN MARKETED WITHOUT THE AMENDMENTS?

By the time Vioxx was approved, concerns had already been raised about the drug's potential to increase heart problems. In the absence of the Amendments, the development timeline would have been shorter. Wouldn't Vioxx have been approved before enough people had been treated with it to alert both regulators and pharmaceutical researchers of its potential problems? Without the Amendments, wouldn't Vioxx have killed even more people?

Although no one can really know the answer, I suspect that Vioxx and other COX-2 inhibitors wouldn't have ever been developed in the absence of the Amendments. Long before the COX-2 enzyme was even discovered, scientists at Upjohn and other laboratories had discovered a way to protect the stomach from the harm caused by stomach acid, anti-inflammatory drugs, and other irritants.

Shortly after I started at Upjohn, my senior colleague, Dr. André Robert, called me to his laboratory to share an exciting discovery. He had been working with prostaglandins in rats and studying their ability to inhibit stomach acid, which seemed to be a necessary condition for the formation of gastric ulcers. Much to his surprise, he had discovered that some prostaglandins could stop ulcer formation by anti-inflammatory agents even at doses that had no effect on stomach acid.

Robert brought me to a laboratory bench where anesthetized rats had been dosed with placebo or micrograms (a very small amount) of prostaglandin before large quantities of indomethacin (an anti-inflammatory drug), alcohol, acid, base, or even boiling water (!) had been put into their stomachs. At autopsy, as expected, rats treated with placebo had bleeding ulcers and inflamed stomachs. Stomachs of rats given very small amounts of prostaglandins, however, had little—if any—damage. Evidently, the prostaglandin could protect the stomach from a variety of irritants even when stomach acid was decreased. Robert called this amazing feat "cytoprotection" (i.e., cell protection) (Robert, Nezamis, Lancaster, et al. 1979, 433–43).

Prostaglandins occur naturally in the stomach and prevent it from being damaged by stomach acid. However, anti-inflammatory drugs stop the formation of those natural hormones; the protection against stomach acid and other irritants, such as alcohol, can be lost. After Robert discovered the cytoprotective properties of the prostaglandins, we tossed around the idea of putting small quantities of them in our ibuprofen products to protect the stomach.

However, the FDA was still resistant to drug combinations (Chapter 3). The agency essentially tripled the amount of regulatory studies required to get such a product on the market by insisting that each component of a combination product, as well as the combination itself, go through toxicology, clinical trials, etc. Had the Amendments not been passed, a combination product might have been feasible.

Such a combination would have likely been much safer than Vioxx, because the prostaglandin would have protected the stomach and been broken down there. Indeed, Robert and his collaborators had identified a cytoprotective prostacyclin derivative that actually inhibited platelet aggregation and that might have protected the heart in the unlikely event that enough of the drug survived and entered the circulatory system (Robert, Aristoff, Wendling, et al. 1985, 619–49). However, largely because of restrictions imposed by the Amendments, Upjohn decided not to develop a cytoprotective prostaglandin.

Although no one can accurately predict a future that hasn't happened, I suspect that other, safer alternatives to Vioxx would have made it to the marketplace without the Amendments. Cytoprotective prostaglandins are only one of the many possibilities that never became available.

The body can be protected from inflammation by omega-3 oils, such as fish oil, without the use of pharmaceuticals. Omega-3 oils are the building blocks of the anti-inflammatory prostaglandins. Aspirin, ibuprofen, and omega-e oils all work on the same pathway, although at different places. However, doctors are often unaware of those alternatives because of restrictions imposed by the Amendments (Chapter 33–34).

We have paid a tremendous cost in both lives and money to implement the Amendments and the legislative bandages that we have applied in an attempt to correct the problems the regulations created (e.g., Waxman-Hatch, Bayer-Doyle, PDFUA). Millions of lives have been lost as the desperately ill wait longer for new drugs, are denied lifesaving information, and lose access to innovations that can no longer be brought to the market profitably. Millions more suffer needlessly, because the drugs that would have increased their mobility, improved their quality of life, or decreased their pain are delayed or totally unavailable.

Pharmaceutical and health care costs have skyrocketed, without any apparent trade-offs in safety. Indeed, all the evidence suggests that the side effects of the Amendments are even more deadly than those of the drugs that they seek to regulate.

... FDA regulation certainly cannot be proved "safe and effective," thereby flunking its own approval criterion.
—Dale H. Gieringer, analyst writing for Cato Institute

Chapter 32

The Amendments Shift Our Medical Paradigm from Prevention to Treatment

An ounce of prevention is worth a pound of cure.
—Benjamin Franklin, Founding Father and scientist

T his chapter details how the Amendments, which were meant to regulate drugs, created a shift from prevention to treatment, along with a loss of life that likely dwarfed the deaths from their negative impact on the pharmaceutical industry. Prevention is a key ingredient in increasing longevity, keeping the quality of life high, and keeping lifetime medical costs low (Goldman, Zheng, Girosi, et al. 2009, 2096–101). When prevention is successful, it lessens, delays, or avoids the need for pharmaceuticals.

In the decade or so before passage of the 1962 Amendments, we were just beginning to appreciate how important nutrition was, not just to prevent overt deficiencies such as rickets and scurvy, but also to maintain optimal health. When I was at Upjohn, we were well aware of the importance of nutrition. Back then, we weren't able to manipulate a laboratory animal's genetics as we are today. Instead, we created disease in the laboratory the old-fashioned way: we changed what we fed our experimental animals.

Our rats and mice were annoyingly healthy. The chow they were given had been packed with all the nutrients that they needed, not just for survival, but also for optimal health. They often didn't develop the diseases that afflicted humans so readily. How could we discover cures for heart disease, gallstones, diabetes, and liver disease if we didn't have animal models with which to test our drugs?

We eventually discovered that if we eliminated certain nutrients from the chow; added excessive sugar, cholesterol, or fat to their diets; or did both, rats and other laboratory animals would develop diseases that look similar to what we saw in humans. Even while we tried to find drugs that would counter those diseases in our animals and—we hoped—in people, many researchers recognized the implications of this dietary manipulation: optimal health depends heavily on optimal nutrition. As a result, those of us in the laboratory exercised and limited our sugar, alcohol, and fat—especially hydrogenated fat—intake. We took vitamin supplements and stayed slim. Our clinical colleagues, who didn't have the everyday experience of trying to produce disease in animals through nutritional manipulation, usually weren't as savvy about lifestyle changes and prevention.

Many of the vitamins necessary for optimal health were made in bulk by pharmaceutical firms. For example, F. Hoffmann–La Roche AG developed processes to produce large quantities of vitamin C and vitamin A; it continues to be a major manufacturer of those and other vitamins (Life Extension Foundation 1994, 86). Merck scientists were the first to purify vitamin B12 (Wegner 2014, 301). Indeed, drug companies were virtually the only places that had the equipment and knowledge to make large quantities of such nutrients. Even today, most supplement manufacturers get their bulk vitamins from pharmaceutical firms.

Not surprisingly, some of the earliest multivitamin supplements were made by the drug industry, such as Upjohn's Unicaps (Figure 5; photo by Hough n.d.) and Bayer's One-A-Day

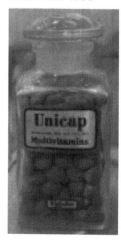

Figure 5. Upjohn's Unicaps Multivitamins circa 1955

Multiple Vitamins. Basically, those supplements were meant to supply the recommended daily allowances (RDAs) of those nutrients. RDAs are the doses necessary to prevent frank vitamin deficiency diseases such as scurvy or rickets. Doses for optimal health are usually considerably higher.

The vitamins in early multivitamin supplements were often synthetic, rather than extracted from natural sources. However, the synthetic vitamins were generally less expensive and could be made in large quantities. In the 1950s and 1960s, before refrigerated trucking was available, people didn't have access to as many fruits and vegetables as we have today. When I was a child in Michigan, our grocery stores had tiny produce sections, which mostly consisted of apples, potatoes, onions, and carrots because those items had a longer shelf life than most other vegetables and fruits. Multivitamins supplied nutrition that might otherwise have been unavailable for a large part of the year.

The pivotal role played by pharmaceutical firms in pioneering the manufacture of vitamins may surprise supplement users today, who generally look with disdain on the pharmaceutical industry. Most people don't realize that many of today's drugs are natural substances that have been chemically modified so that their action is prolonged, their absorption is better, their structure allows them to be patented, or a combination of those attributes. The Amendments have made this last criterion an all-important one.

Many people interested in nutrition believe that natural products can't be patented. That actually isn't the case. The problem with natural products is that information about their structure and function is usually published long before someone thinks of patenting them. If a patent on the structure or use of any chemical—natural or artificial—isn't filed within a certain amount of time after such disclosures, they are forever in the public domain (i.e., become unpatentable). Once this occurs, even a "use patent" for such a product becomes more problematic.

For example, prostaglandins of the E and F families have structures complex enough that they were never disclosed before the patent filing.

Consequently, the US patent office issued a patent even though the prostaglandins were naturally occurring hormones (US Patent 1962).

As the development process became more expensive, companies could no longer stay solvent while taking unpatentable products through the FDA's regulatory process. This was not always the case. Shortly after I joined the Upjohn Company in the mid-1970s, management instructed the research departments to stop proposing unpatentable drugs for development. Increased emphasis was put on projections of earnings before deciding to put money and time into development. In the first few years that I was with the company, concern about patentability and market projections went from a consideration to a primary precondition for development.

Chapter 33

Expensive Drugs Are Now Replacing Affordable Natural Products

The Amendment-driven need for patent protection necessitated the development of expensive new drugs as a substitute for widely available, inexpensive alternatives. For example, at one time the Upjohn Company was developing a series of antioxidants that were nicknamed "lazeroids" (after Lazarus, the biblical individual brought back to life by Jesus Christ). The lazeroids seemed to improve the outcome in a wide variety of diseases.

While traveling, I was approached by an ailing gentleman who had heard of the lazeroids and wanted to try them even though they were not yet fully tested or FDA approved. I contacted the head of the project and asked if this was possible. "We can't give him the lazeroids at this point in the development process," I was told. "Just tell him to take lots of vitamin E; it will do the same thing."

If vitamin E would do the same thing, why was my employer developing lazeroids? The answer was quite simple. The development program for either compound would have cost close to the same in money and in time. However, we had patent protection on the lazeroids and therefore had a chance of recovering our development costs. Had we proceeded with vitamin E, generic manufacturers would have been able to promote their product with a much-abbreviated expense.

Consequently, it was unlikely that we would ever be able to recover development costs.

The reader might justifiably wonder why vitamin E manufacturers couldn't simply let both doctors and patients know how beneficial it was without going through the development process. After all, vitamin E isn't what we normally think of as a drug.

The Amendments charged the FDA with making sure that every drug had "substantial evidence" of effectiveness. If companies advertise that their products can help treat disease, the FDA considers those products to be drugs even if they are normally thought of as food or vitamins. The FDA generally accepts as substantial evidence only studies that have been conducted under its costly regulatory umbrella. A company selling nutrients risks FDA seizure of its inventory and criminal prosecution if it claims that a nutritional product can treat disease, *even if that claim is well-documented*!

Chapter 34

The Amendments Are Responsible for the "American Thalidomide"

ronically, the Amendments, which were intended to prevent tragedies like thalidomide, actually caused what I refer to as the "American thalidomide." In the early 1980s, several reports in medical journals indicated that the B vitamin, folic acid, taken early in pregnancy could prevent a number of birth defects (Smithells, Sheppard, Schorah, et al. 1981, 911–18).

Supplementing with 800 micrograms almost completely inhibited debilitating neural tube defects, such as spina bifida (Czeizel 1992, 1832–35). Naturally, folic acid manufacturers wished to advertise this incredible benefit of their product. However, the FDA deemed that such a claim made this B-vitamin a drug. Folic acid would have go through the expensive drug development process if the manufacturers wished to advertise its benefits to America's young women.

In 1992, the Centers for Disease Control (CDC), another government agency, began recommending that women of childbearing age take folic acid supplements because their protective effects were required as supplementation during the first 6 weeks of pregnancy (Milunsky, H Jick, SS Jick, et al. 1989, 2847–52) when a young woman might not be aware of her condition. The FDA warned folic acid manufacturers not to even refer to the Center's recommendation, because this action would be considered illegal advertising (Palca 1992, 1857; Tabarrok 2000, 25–53; Calfee 1997). Instead of manufacturers paying to inform the American public about folic acid, taxpayers had to do so through the CDC.

Advertising is a primary way in which many people, especially the poor, receive new medical information. The poor see their doctors much less frequently than do the affluent, and they get much of their medical information from advertising on television or elsewhere. Had folic acid manufacturers been permitted to advertise their products in print, on television, and on the radio, many more young women would have been aware of this inexpensive preventative.

In 1995, the Netherlands started exactly this kind of mass media campaign to educate young women about the importance of supplementing with folic acid. In just 3 years, the proportion of women using folic acid during pregnancy increased from 8% to 63% (De Walle, Van der Pal, De Jong-Van den Berg, et al. 1998, 826–27; De Walle, De Jong-Van den Berg, & Cornel 1999, 1187). Had US folic acid manufacturers been permitted to advertise the benefits of their product back in the 1980s, we might have seen an increase in supplementation in the United States—and a decline in birth defects.

Instead, approximately 10,000 American babies were born with deformities more horrific than those caused by thalidomide.[23] Thousands more were aborted, because neural tube and other birth defects are tested for prenatally. The American thalidomide incident has been even more tragic than the European one, because it could have been easily avoided. *The Amendments caused birth defects in American babies instead of preventing them.*

The FDA clearly knew that folic acid was effective in preventing birth defects, even though it wouldn't allow folic acid manufacturers to share this knowledge. In 1998, the agency began requiring grain products to be supplemented with folic acid (US FDA 1996, 8781–97). Unfortunately, fortification does not ensure that young women are getting the dose required to protect their babies from crippling birth defects. The FDA refused to allow folic acid manufacturers to make the claim that "800 micrograms of folic acid is more effective in reducing the risk of neural tube defects than a lower amount in common food form," even when the agency was twice directed by the courts to do so (see Chapter 37).

Today, most physicians will recommend folic acid supplements to their pregnant patients. However, because supplementation is needed in the first two months after conception, the damage may already be done by the time a woman goes to her doctor to confirm a pregnancy. Prohibiting manufacturers from advertising the benefits of folic acid in the mass media for almost two decades meant that children who could have been born healthy were aborted or born with crippling injuries.

Chapter 35

Information about Nutrition Is a Matter of Life and Death

F
olic acid is only one example of how the Amendments, as interpreted by the FDA, have muzzled manufacturers of vitamins, foods, and other forms of nutritional support, thereby sentencing the American public to debilitating diseases that might otherwise have been prevented. Indeed, I suspect that Amendment-driven suppression of this information has been more deadly than all of the other side effects of the Amendments described so far.

The word "vitamin" comes from the Latin word "vita," meaning life. Vitamins are necessary for life; we cannot survive without them. In most cases, the human body can't make those critical nutrients or can't make them in sufficient quantities, so the body deteriorates. Most vitamins were first discovered when their deficiencies caused severe health problems, which were reversed or prevented by supplementation with the critical nutrient.

For example, as Europeans migrated from the farms into the cities during the Industrial Revolution, their children developed the crippling bone disease known as rickets. By the early 20th century, more than 80% of children in North America and Europe suffered from it. Along the coasts of Britain and Scandinavia, parents gave their offspring cod liver oil without knowing that it contained the hormone we now call vitamin D, which prevented the dreaded disease.

Rickets can also be treated with or prevented by sunlight or, today, by artificial ultraviolet (UV) light (Holick 2005, 2739S–48S), which helps our skin make vitamin D. However, people living in far northern or southern countries usually can't get enough sunlight in the winter to produce optimal levels of vitamin D. Even though we fortify many foods with vitamin D today, most people in those countries are deficient in this critical vitamin—and suffer the consequences.

Vitamin D deficiency is now recognized as an epidemic in the United States.
—Dr. Michael F. Holick, Vitamin D Laboratory, Boston University School of Medicine

Like most vitamins, vitamin D doesn't affect just one part of the body. Every day, we are discovering how important vitamins, minerals, and other natural substances are to optimal health. Most Americans, however, are unaware of those discoveries, because manufacturers risk bankruptcy and criminal prosecution if they inform the public about some of the new findings. Most people are unaware that the recommended daily allowances (RDAs) of vitamins and minerals might prevent overt disease, but that much larger amounts of those nutrients are necessary for optimal health.

For example, when Finnish infants are not supplemented with vitamin D in their first year of birth, almost five times as many develop Type I (insulin-dependent) diabetes than do the infants who received 2,000 I.U. (Hypponen, Laara, Reunanen, et al. 2001, 1500–03). Type I diabetes is thought to be an auto-immune disorder, so it's not surprising that vitamin D might protect against other auto-immune diseases, such as multiple sclerosis (MS). Children born to mothers with high vitamin D levels appear to have a lower risk of MS, for example (Simon, Munger, & Ascherio 2012, 246–51). When 187,000 American women took 400 IU or more of vitamin D daily, their children had a 41% reduction of MS over the next 10 to 20 years (Munger, Zhang, O'Reilly, et al. 2004, 60–65).

Although Type II diabetes is not generally considered an autoimmune disorder, supplementing adult women with both vitamin D and calcium reduces the incidence of Type II diabetes in high-risk populations by 33% (Pittas, Dawson-Hughes, Li, et al. 2006, 650–56; Pittas, Lau, Hu, et al. 2007, 2017–29). Apparently, vitamin D also influences the action of insulin (Borissova, Tankova, Kirilov, et al. 2003, 258–56).

Diabetic patients have 2.3 times as many medical costs compared to those of the average person: $176 Billion in 2012, in addition to $69 billion in disability, lost work, and premature death (Yang, Dall, Halder, et al. 2013, 1033–46). Slashing diabetes with low-cost vitamin D and calcium supplementation could save billions of dollars, but the FDA forbids supplement manufacturers to share this information with the American public, courtesy of the Amendments.

People in northern latitudes receive less sunshine than people living closer to the equator do; their blood levels of vitamin D are lower too. The rate of heart problems increases with low vitamin D levels (Patrycja, León de la Fuente, Nilsen, et al. 2013; Zittermann, Schleithoff, & Koerfer 2005, 483–92; Wang 2013), as does cancer incidence (Ng 2014, 339–45). A child carried by a vitamin D–deficient mother is at greater risk to developing both diabetes and cardiovascular disease as an adult (Stene, Ulriksen, Magnus, et al. 2000, 1093–98; Lucas, Ponsonby, Pasco, et al. 2008, 710–20).

An estimated 20–80% of United States, Canadian, and European men and women are vitamin D deficient (Ganji, Zhang, & Tangpricha 2012, 498–507; Greene-Finestone, Berger, de Groh, et al. 2011, 1389–99; Gonzalez-Gross, Valtuena, Breidenassel, et al. 2012, 755–64). People with low blood levels of vitamin D (less than 15 ng/ml) are more than twice as likely to have a heart attack than are those with higher levels (greater than 30 ng/ml) (Giovannucci, Liu, Hollis, et al. 2008, 1174–80). People ages 50–79 with lower levels of vitamin D in their blood have a 57% greater risk of dying, primarily from cardiovascular disease (Schöttker, Jorde, Peasey, et al. 2014, g3656). Vitamin D levels greater than 30 ng/ml result in a 75% decrease in deaths from all causes and a 67% reduction in cardiovascular deaths (Thomas, Hartaigh, Bosch, et al. 2012, 1158–64).

Because cardiovascular disease is the number one killer in the developed world, many lives could be saved if people understood how important it is to maintain sufficient blood levels of this particular vitamin. For example, Dr. William B. Grant, former NASA physicist and current director of Sunlight, Nutrition, and Health Research Center, estimated that low vitamin D levels might contribute to as much as 60% of disease world-wide. He believes that doubling the blood levels of this vitamin might add about 2 years to the average world-wide life expectancy (Grant 2011, 1016–26), saving about 400,000 Americans from premature death each year alone (Grant 2009, 207–14).

However, not all studies show benefits with vitamin D supplementation. Like most biological molecules, vitamin D's interaction with the body is complex. How people respond to vitamin D supplementation can depend on their genetic heritage (Carlberg, Seuter, de Mello, et al. 2013, e71042; Morand, da Silva, Hier, et al. 2014, 309). Protection against heart disease, cancer, and bone loss requires different blood levels of the vitamin (Spedding, Vanlint, Morris, et al. 2013, 5127–39). The length of treatment appears to be important too: one researcher reviewing published studies indicated that a 3-year supplementation with vitamin D protected people against all-cause mortality, but shorter durations of the supplementation did not (Zheng, Zhu, Zhou, et al. 2013, e82109). The level of calcium (Liu, Prescott, Giovannucci, et al. 2013, 1411–17) and perhaps other nutrients influences how effective vitamin D is. In other words, just like pharmaceuticals, nutritional supplements don't always work the same way in everyone.

Your doctor may not be aware of the research about vitamin D, because the vitamin manufacturers are legally forbidden from sharing this information directly with doctors. Unlike the pharmaceutical representatives, firms marketing vitamins cannot visit doctors' offices and educate them about the lifesaving benefits of the products. Because such visits are, for many busy physicians, the primary way that they learn about new scientific developments, the Amendments greatly delay—and sometimes prevent—the incorporation of lifesaving natural products into medical practice. If, as Grant estimated, we are each losing years of life simply because the Amendments don't allow physicians to easily gain knowledge about vitamin D, imagine how many years of life we are losing because our doctors are usually unaware of the lifesaving effects of other vitamins and minerals!

In many cases, such natural products could substitute for pharmaceuticals with fewer side effects. If the Amendments were not responsible for inflating development costs approximately 40-fold (Chapter 19), drug companies would likely have continued research on vitamins, minerals, and other natural products and sold them profitably by educating both the public and medical profession about them.

Determining how many lives have been lost because of the Amendment-driven restrictions that the FDA put on nutritional information detailed in the past couple of chapters and the ones following is not easy. If Grant is right about vitamin D supplementation giving each person about 2 more years of life, it's likely that each of us would gain many more years of life if information for all vitamins, minerals, and other supplements were more available. Indeed, given how the Amendments distorted the drug industry, interfered with the practice of medicine, and suppressed lifesaving information about supplements, it's not difficult to see how we've all likely lost years of our lives to the Amendments.

Chapter 36

The Amendments Restrict Information about Prevention

The First Amendment to the US Constitution guarantees the right of free speech, but the FDA claims that that right does not apply to commercial speech. If you sell a product, the FDA forbids you to advertise its health benefits or disease prevention without going through the expensive and time-consuming approval process. Any health claim by a manufacturer turns a food (see Chapters 38–39), vitamin, or supplement into a drug in the eyes of the FDA. As I once testified as an expert witness in court, by this logic, a company selling water could not advertise that it alleviated dehydration without going through years of expensive studies to demonstrate what is obvious and already well-established.

Looked at from a narrow regulatory standpoint, the FDA is simply trying to be consistent. Upjohn, for example, discovered that its blood pressure–lowering medication, minoxidil, had a highly desirable side effect. Balding men who took the product found that their hair started growing back. After much debate about whether Upjohn should start making cosmetic as well as therapeutic products, the company gained FDA approval for prescription Rogaine®, a topical minoxidil solution, to partially reverse the balding process.

Shortly after Rogaine was marketed in 1988, another company began advertising a mixture of nutrients to re-grow hair on the balding scalp.

Upjohn management thought about suing the other company, but decided against it. Why did Upjohn have to spend millions of dollars and
years of time before it could sell a product to stimulate hair growth, while
the other company need not jump through those regulatory hoops?

Clearly, the other company could justifiably argue that the mixture of
nutrients wouldn't be expected to have safety problems. However, safety
wasn't the primary issue; thanks to the Amendments, effectiveness claims
were. The FDA designates any product making a health claim as a drug
to avoid having a system where drugs have to go through an expensive
regulatory process and nutritional products do not. As we'll discuss in
Chapter 37, the courts have agreed with the FDA.

Because of the sheer volume of information and the number of manufacturers, however, the FDA has a difficult time enforcing its restrictions.
Moreover, as we'll see in Chapter 36, when the FDA makes an example of
a company or individual, the agency does so in a way that could be con-
strued as cruel and unusual punishment. Others who might be tempted
to share lifesaving information are effectively discouraged from doing so.

I certainly was intimidated by my knowledge of FDA tactics when I
invented a cream to prevent skin damage from radiation treatments for cancer. In 2003, I was diagnosed with ductal carcinoma in situ of the breast.
Whole breast radiation treatment was recommended, and I opted to have it.

In my orientation visit about a week before receiving radiation, I discovered that women already being treated had weeping sores on their
breasts. This concerned me greatly because my skin is easily damaged by
the sun's radiation. Although the radiation given to cancer patients is of
a different type, it was likely that my skin would be sensitive to this kind
of radiation as well.

Radiation damage results in inflammation of the skin, which, of
course, involves pro-inflammatory prostaglandins. If I could give my skin
the building blocks for anti-inflammatory prostaglandins, maybe I could
protect it. I put together a cream with various nutrients, figuring that the
skin would use what it needed and ignore the rest. Mother Nature, after
all, has given us bodies that exhibit a great deal of inherent wisdom.

I had no time to test the cream before my treatment, so I erred on the side of including everything that I thought the skin might need. Every component was sold as a nutritional supplement; I added no drugs, prescription products, or chemically altered substances.

Given the haste with which I put the cream together and the lack of testing, I was surprised when the cream actually worked. The final few treatments left me with a tan but no burning or open sores. The doctor made a notation in my chart indicating that the cream had likely been responsible for my good results; he indicated even after a single month of treatment, he couldn't tell which breast received radiation.

Thankful for having been able to protect myself, I offered to give some cream to my doctor for patients who might want to try it. He told me he would like some but only after I got FDA approval for it. Clearly, he feared that he could get in trouble offering patients something that hadn't been through the regulatory hoops.

A few weeks later, my neighbor came home from visiting her parents in another state. She had accidentally burned herself with caramelized sugar while baking. She had second-degree burns on her wrist that had persisted for days. Her own doctor couldn't see her for another week. She was in pain and asked me if I was aware of anything that might give her temporary relief.

I told her that I wasn't a medical doctor, so I couldn't advise her. I did, however, give her some of my cream; it didn't have anything in it that should cause harm. If the cream actually worked the way I had designed it, her pain might at least partially subside.

The next day she stopped by. Not only had the cream alleviated her pain, but also new skin covered the burn except for a small spot that she claimed didn't get any cream. She wanted to try the cream to heal her face, which had been scarred by a laser peel gone awry several years earlier.

The body replaces many cells quickly, but scars "turn over" quite slowly. I gave her 6 months worth of cream to be used twice daily. Remarkably, by the time she had used up the cream, she told me that about 80% of her scarring was gone.

I realized that the American public might benefit from such a product. Of course, to market it for preventing radiation burn, healing burns, or reversing scarring, I would need to go through the FDA's development program. To get investors (I was no longer with the pharmaceutical industry), I'd need a patent, so I hired a friend of mine who was a patent attorney to take the cream through the patenting process.

As she requested, I sent her a sample. As she was putting together the claims, she called to ask me if the cream might help heal her dermatomyo-fibromas, which are small benign growths on the skin. She went to a surgeon regularly to have them removed. Her next appointment was scheduled a few days later.

All I could really tell her is that the cream didn't have anything in it that should make her condition worse. She called me two days later to tell me that she had cancelled her doctor's appointment because the dermatomyo-fibromas were gone. She included this information in the patent application (US Patent 2008).

As we'll see in the next chapter, the FDA doesn't always look favorably on inventors using natural products to deal with medical issues. Indeed, the agency generally treats innovators as criminals, guilty of quackery until proven innocent. My knowledge of their tactics certainly had a chilling effect on my natural desire to share the cream with those who might benefit.

Chapter 37

The FDA Raids Stores and Physicians Promoting Prevention

The Food and Drug Administration is charged by Congress with an onerous responsibility—that of protecting the nation's health. Instead of shouldering this heavy responsibility, we find the agency engaged in bizarre games of cops and robbers. Instead of a guardian of the national health, we find an agency which is police-oriented, chiefly concerned with prosecutions and convictions, totally indifferent to individuals' rights, and bent on using snooping gear to pry and invade citizens' right of privacy.
—Senator Edward V. Long, Hearing of the Senate Subcommittee on Administrative Practice and Procedure, 1965

HEALTH FOOD STORES IN TEXAS

Between 1992 and 1993, the FDA—in collaboration with other state and federal agencies—raided 52 Texas health food stores, seizing products such as flaxseed oil, aloe vera, zinc supplements, vitamin C, Sleepytime Tea, and nutritional products designed by Dr. Kurt Donsabch and Dr. Hans Neiper. Sometimes SWAT teams descended on the stores as if their employees were armed criminals. Homes of owners and employees were sometimes raided as well.

During the 8 years I was an investigator with the Texas Attorney General's Office, I had numerous occasions to work with the FDA on cases involving potential health fraud. I repeatedly saw cases against large corporations ... go unchallenged.... [I]nstead, the agency chose (to pursue) cases against alternative health care providers and minor companies.... Chinese herbalists, health food stores, and chiropractors were among their favorite targets....
—Marion Moss, former investigator, Texas Attorney General's office, writing in *New Times*, Seattle, Washington, 1992

The confiscated products were never returned, no charges were filed, and no justification for the raids was given. The raids were likely intended simply to be disruptive to those selling products that the FDA frowned upon (Adams 2007).

TAHOMA CLINIC, TAHOMA, WASHINGTON

On May 6, 1992, armed local police officers and FDA agents raided the clinic of Dr. Jonathan Wright, one of the country's foremost nutritional doctors. For 14 hours, agents terrorized patients, employees, and the doctor. They seized patient records, computers, vitamin supplies, and various natural therapy products.

Agents then went to the homes of patients and employees to interrogate them about the clinic's practices. Wright was never charged with a crime. The FDA assumes that alternative medical practitioners make claims about vitamins and minerals, turning those products into illegal drugs (Williams 1992).

Wright filed suit against the FDA, claiming violations of the physician–patient privilege and unreasonable intrusion into his medical practice. In retaliation, the FDA announced its intentions to examine confiscated medical records of more than 50 patients. In December 1992, Judge John Weinberg ruled that those records must be given to the court instead (Adams 2007). Years later, Wright got a portion of his records and property back.

The time, expense, and disruption involved here are enormous. It quite obviously will interfere with our ability to deliver the best possible health care to those who come to see us. Perhaps that is the point.
—Dr. Jonathan Wright, commenting on the raids

Wright is one of my trusted medical advisors. Without his vast knowledge of nutrition, some of my health problems could have turned into real-life nightmares. He is perhaps best known for developing bio-identical HRT (hormone replacement therapy) (Morgenthaler & Wright 1997; Wright & Lenard 2009), as popularized by Suzanne Somers (Somers & Greene 2005). Had the raid destroyed Wright's practice, untold women would have been denied a safer and more flexible alternative to pharmaceutical HRT, which has been shown to be carcinogenic (Lyytinen, Pukkala, & Ylikorkala 2009, 65–73).

THE LIFE EXTENSION FOUNDATION, FORT LAUDERDALE, FLORIDA

The Life Extension Foundation (LEF) has a long history of informing consumers about the benefits of vitamins and other natural products, as well as drugs that are marketed overseas but are not available in the United States. The FDA looks on such information as selling or recommending unapproved drugs. Coenzyme Q10 (CoQ10), which will be discussed in Chapter 39, was one of the targets of the seizure (Faloon 2015, 7–15, esp. 12–13).

On February 6, 1987, the FDA sent a couple of dozen agents and US Marshalls to the LEF's warehouse and store, where they smashed the glass doors and entered with guns drawn. They confiscated products, 5,000 copies of LEF's magazine, computers, and even personal effects. Only 20% of the seized items were covered under the warrant. The FDA agent who supplied information for it later confessed to falsifying information. Property of another tenant in the building was also illegally seized.

LEF consulted multiple attorneys, who advised LEF's founders, Bill Faloon and Saul Kent, that they were looking at 5–20 years in prison unless they plea-bargained. They were told that they couldn't win against the FDA with its taxpayer-supplied attorneys. Undaunted, Faloon and Kent stood their ground and fought back against the 28-count criminal indictment. Nine years after the initial raid, the last count against them was dismissed.

LEF spent about $1.3 million in its defense. This cost was almost the same amount of money that LEF had been putting into life extension research at that time. The time and money spent fighting the FDA could have been channeled instead to studies that could have lengthened our lives. The FDA probably spent more than $1.3 million in taxpayer dollars to stop LEF from informing us about how nutrients and drugs could help us live longer lives (Kent 1996).

LEF has a long history of being on the forefront of information about nutrients and drugs available only outside the United States (LEF 2015). I have been a customer for decades and have learned a great deal from LEF's thoughtful reviews, which document the science behind the statements. LEF took the lead on educating Americans about the benefits of vitamin D supplementation. Had the FDA been successful in jailing LEF's founders, a great deal of lifesaving information would have been unavailable to most Americans for years, perhaps even decades.

Unfortunately, LEF's case was not unusual. Both Wright and LEF documented more than 24 raids on other nutritionally based companies—including those that supplied vitamin chows for pets—which usually ended in bankrupting the owners or landing them in jail after a plea-bargain. Even in the few cases where supplement manufacturers prevailed, they did so at great cost (Kent 1994; Wright 1992).

… the fact that the FDA is willing to jail its political opponents sends a chilling message to pioneering doctors and scientists [who] were seeking to make major medical advances available to dying Americans.
—"The FDA Suffers Another Legal Defeat," *Life Extension Magazine*, October 1999

Chapter 38

The FDA Refuses to Obey Courts Orders

If the Food and Drug Administration would spend a little less time and effort on small manufacturers of vitamins and milk substitutes and a little more on the large manufacturers of ... dangerous drugs ... the public would be better served.
—Senator Edward V. Long, in the 1965 Hearing of the Senate Subcommittee on Administrative Practice and Procedure

After the passage of the Amendments, the FDA made several unsuccessful attempts to bring nutritional supplements under its regulatory umbrella. In 1962, the FDA tried to set minimum and maximum potency levels for dietary supplements but backed off because of strong public protest. In 1965, the FDA published a rule (regulation) that any dietary supplement exceeding 150% of the RDA for a vitamin or mineral would be regulated as a drug and could not be sold without FDA drug approval. Senator William Proxmire introduced an amendment that prohibited the FDA from classifying a vitamin or a mineral as a drug based on its potency. The FDA made several attempts to get around this provision without success, because of a backlash from both the public and the courts (Emord 2006).

The FDA … (is) actively hostile against the manufacture, sale, and distribution of vitamins and minerals as food or food supplements. They are out to get the health food industry and drive the health food stores out of business. And they are trying to do this out of active hostility and prejudice.
—Senator William Proxmire, *National Health Federation Bulletin*, April 1974

The effectiveness provision of the Amendments finally gave the FDA a way to indirectly regulate the sharing of health information about nutritional supplements. Manufacturers could say very little about their products; consumers had to rely on getting information from other sources.

In an attempt to remedy this situation, Congress passed the Nutrition Labeling and Education Act of 1990 (NLEA), which would allow nutrient manufacturers to make claims once the FDA established a review procedure. The FDA ended up rejecting most claims.

Concerned citizens joined with supplement manufacturers to sue the FDA on the grounds that the agency's stringent requirements created an unconstitutional restriction on free speech. Specifically, the suit focused on four claims: that antioxidants may reduce cancer risk, that fiber consumption may reduce colorectal cancer risk, that omega-3 fatty acids may reduce heart disease, and that 800 micrograms of folic acid in a dietary supplement is more effective in reducing neural tube defects than is a lower amount in foods.

The FDA balks at any attempt to share such information with consumers, for fear this evidence will harm the drug industry. After all, the PDUFA user fees cover most of the numerous personnel hired to speed approvals.

… the task force considered many issues in its deliberations including to ensure that the existence of dietary supplements on the market does not act as disincentive for drug development.…
—FDA Dietary Supplements Task Force Final Report, June 1992

In January 1999, the US District Court for the District of Columbia ruled on an appeal against the FDA and ordered it to construct disclaimers to add the plaintiffs' folic acid labels if the FDA really thought they were misleading. The courts also instructed the FDA to give manufacturers clearer guidance as to what it considered "significant scientific agreement," its standard for evaluation of claims (US District Court for DC 1999).

In November 2000, the plaintiffs sued again, because the FDA had not done as instructed. After hearing the arguments, the court concluded that "the agency appears to have at best, misunderstood, and at worst, deliberately ignored, highly relevant portions of the Court of Appeals Opinion." The court remanded the folic acid claim to FDA with instructions that the agency draft one or more "short, succinct, and accurate alternative disclaimers, which may be chosen by Plaintiffs to accompany their Folic Acid Claim"(US District Court for DC 1999).

The FDA continued to use our tax dollars to appeal those cases (Emord 2006). In January 2004, the US District Court for the District of Columbia on appeal finally sided with the FDA's argument that making claims to treat a disease, as opposed to preventing the disorder, converted any food or supplement into a drug (US Court 2004). Consequently, the FDA began sending out warning letters to food producers, as described in the next chapter.

Chapter 39

The FDA Turns Foods into Drugs

S hoppers rarely know how the FDA influences what food producers can tell them. The objections in the "warning letters" are at
times so unbelievable that I've quoted them at length and bolded
sections where the FDA indicates that such foods are considered to be
pharmaceuticals.

CHERRY GROWERS

The FDA sent warning letters to 29 producers of cherries and cherry
products in 2005. An example of the text of those letters is as follows:

The labeling for your cherry products on your website bears
the following claims:

"[C]herries may have the potential to

- relieve arthritis pain and inflammation …

- inhibit the growth of certain cancers

[L]ab tests show that the anthocyanins in red tart cherries give
10 times the anti-inflammatory relief of aspirin, without irri-
tating the stomach …"

This list of claims is not intended to be all-inclusive, but represents the types of claims found in your product labeling. **These claims cause your products to be drugs … a new drug may not be legally marketed in the United States without an approved New Drug Application (NDA)** (US FDA 2005b).

A drug requires an NDA, which is the literal truckload of data containing the FDA-mandated studies that take more than a decade to produce and cost more than a billion out-of-pocket dollars (see Chapters 6 and 17, respectively). Clearly, such time and money is beyond what farmers and their associations would be able to spend to make FDA-approved health claims.

CHEERIOS MANUFACTURERS

The FDA sent the manufacturer of this popular cereal a warning letter on May 5, 2009, that included the following language:

Based on claims made on your product's label, we have determined that your **Cheerios® Toasted Whole Grain Oat Cereal is promoted for conditions that cause it to be a drug** because the product is intended for use in the prevention, mitigation, and treatment of disease. Specifically, your Cheerios® product bears the following claims on its label:

- "Did you know that in just 6 weeks Cheerios can reduce bad cholesterol by an average of 4 percent? Cheerios is … clinically proven to lower cholesterol. A clinical study showed that eating two 1 1/2 cup servings daily of Cheerios cereal reduced bad cholesterol when eaten as part of a diet low in saturated fat and cholesterol."

These claims indicate that Cheerios® is intended for use in lowering cholesterol and, therefore, in preventing, mitigating, and treating the disease hypercholesterolemia (US FDA 2009).

WALNUT DISTRIBUTORS

On February 22, 2010, the FDA sent a warning letter to Diamond Foods concerning its advertising material for walnuts. An excerpt from the letter includes the following language:

Based on claims made on your firm's website, we have determined that **your walnut products are promoted for conditions that cause them to be drugs** because these products are intended for use in the prevention, mitigation, and treatment of disease. The following are examples of the claims made on your firm's website under the heading of a web page stating "OMEGA-3s ... Every time you munch a few walnuts, you're doing your body a big favor."

• "Studies indicate that the omega-3 fatty acids found in walnuts may help lower cholesterol; protect against heart disease, stroke, and some cancers; ease arthritis and other inflammatory diseases; and even fight depression and other mental illnesses."

• "[O]mega-3 fatty acids inhibit the tumor growth that is promoted by the acids found in other fats ... "

• "[I]n treating major depression, for example, omega-3s seem to work by making it easier for brain cell receptors to process mood-related signals from neighboring neurons."

• "The omega-3s found in fish oil are thought to be responsible for the significantly lower incidence of breast cancer in Japanese women as compared to women in the United States."

Because of these intended uses, your walnut products are drugs within the meaning of section 201 (g)(1)(B) of the Act [21 U.S.C. § 321(g)(B)]. Your walnut products are also new drugs under section 201(p) of the Act [21 U.S.C. § 321(p)] because **they are not generally recognized as safe and effective for the above referenced conditions.** Therefore, under section 505(a) of the Act [21 U.S.C. § 355(a)], they may not be legally marketed with the above claims in the United States without an approved new drug application. **Additionally, your walnut products are offered for conditions that are not amenable to self-diagnosis and treatment by individuals who are not medical practitioners; therefore, adequate directions for use cannot be written so that a layperson can use these drugs safely for their intended purposes. Thus, your walnut products are also misbranded** under section 502(f)(1) of the Act, in that the labeling for these drugs fails to bear adequate directions for use [21 U.S.C. § 352(f)(1)]" (US FDA 2010b).

Largely on the basis of the FDA's letter, a class action suit was brought against Diamond Foods for false advertising. Diamond settled out-of-court for $2.6 million (Goldstein, Edelstein, & Roth 2012). That's a high price to pay for letting customers know about the health benefits of walnuts.

Notice that the FDA is not claiming that cherries, Cheerios®, or walnuts will harm those who eat them or are contaminated. The agency is claiming that telling people about a food's health benefits—including the findings of published scientific studies—turns a food into a drug. Such wording therefore becomes a crime unless the manufacturer goes through the same approval process that a drug does!

Because we die if we don't eat, it's pretty obvious that food can have a health impact. When scientific studies define the details of this impact, and when manufacturers quote the details, the FDA believes that those foods become drugs and must jump through their regulatory hoops.

Chapter 40

Supplements Make Drugs Safer

STATINS AND COQ10

Any drug or nutrient that decreases cardiovascular disease adds many years to our lives. Statins, for example, reduce the risk of major coronary events, such as heart attacks, by 31% and death from all causes by 21% (LaRosa, He, & Sjama 1999, 2340–46). Although statins were developed to lower bad cholesterol, they are thought to work primarily by lowering inflammation responsible for the buildup of plaque in the coronary arteries (Jain & Ridker 2005, 977–87).

The body makes Coenzyme Q10 (CoQ10), which aids in energy production. When combined with statins, CoQ10 supplementation decreases strokes and heart attacks in the first year compared with statins alone (Singh, Neki, Kartikey, et al. 2003, 75–82; Mortensen, Rosenfeldt, Kumar, et al. 2014, 641–49). Patients taking statins supplemented with CoQ10 for 2 years had 44% fewer deaths than did those not taking CoQ10, both from cardiovascular events and from all causes (Mortensen, Rosenfeldt, Kumar, et al. 2014). CoQ10, while effective on its own, also enhances the lifesaving effects of statins.

This result isn't surprising, because some of the side effects of statins are due to the depletion of CoQ10, which is made by the same pathway as cholesterol. Consequently, long-term usage depletes CoQ10, thereby resulting in a condition called myopathy, or muscle weakness. Muscles need CoQ10 to function properly, so administering CoQ10 along with statins prevents this serious side effect (Zlatohlavek, Vrablik, Grauova, et al. 2012, 98–101). Indeed, the fatigue resulting from statins is reduced from 41% to 7% in patients taking this supplement (Singh, Neki, Kartikey, et al. 2003).

Clearly, CoQ10—by itself or combined with statins—offers great promise to patients with heart disease. The FDA, however, tried to outlaw this lifesaving supplement. CoQ10 was sold as a prescription drug in Japan, so the FDA felt this natural product should be sold in the United States as a prescription drug too. The agency seized CoQ10 products from several suppliers, including twice from LEF (Faloon 2004), claiming that talking about the cardiovascular benefits of CoQ10 made it a drug that had to go through the expensive and time-consuming drug development process before Americans could buy it.

Because CoQ10 is such an important part of our body's biochemistry, its benefits are likely to go beyond heart disease. Indeed, CoQ10 appears to have anti-cancer properties as well (Lockwood, Moesgaard, Hanioka, et al. 1994, S231–40; Lockwood, Moesgaard, Yamamoto, et al. 1995, 172–77; Premkumar, Yuvaraj, Vijayasarathy, et al. 2007, 367–70; Lockwood, Moesgaard, & Folkers 1994, 1504–08). Had the FDA been successful in limiting access to CoQ10, many more American lives would have been lost.

ACETAMINOPHEN AND N-ACETYL CYSTEINE

In its wisdom, the body breaks down drugs and other foreign substances so that they don't build up to dangerous levels. In the process, large amounts of precious nutrients are often consumed. Although the body usually has sufficient stores of most nutrients to detoxify a single drug dose, our storehouse of nutrients can be depleted with chronic medications. When the body doesn't have enough nutrients to detoxify drugs and maintain body function, the organs that detoxify drugs, primarily the liver and kidney, can be harmed.

The over-the-counter drug, acetaminophen, for example, consumes the naturally occurring antioxidant, glutathione, as the drug is broken down in the liver. Acetaminophen is the active ingredient in Tylenol and in about 600 other drugs (KnowYourDose.org 2017). Too great a depletion of glutathione results in liver damage severe enough to cause death.

Acetaminophen overdose, about half of which is accidental (Baniasadi, Eftekhari, Tabarsi, et al. 2010, 1235–38), is treated by giving large doses of N-acetyl cysteine, a natural product that stimulates more glutathione production (Yarema, Johnson, Berlin, et al. 2009, 606–14). An estimated 458 Americans die each year from acetaminophen-induced liver failure, 2,600 patients are hospitalized, and 56,000 are treated in the emergency room (Lee 2004, 6–9). Most accidental poisonings happen when the liver's glutathione and other antioxidants have already been depleted by the person's drinking or taking other drugs that are detoxified by the liver.

Because both N-acetyl cysteine and acetaminophen can be bought separately without a prescription, combining them into one pill to make a safer pain reliever would save lives. The FDA, however, would not allow such combination products on the market without extensive, time-consuming, and costly studies of each component, plus the combination. Because the combination is too obvious to be patented, it's unlikely that a company could recover its development costs. Because so many over-the-counter products contain acetaminophen, accidental overdoses, which could be easily and inexpensively prevented, are likely to continue thanks to the Amendments.

Chapter 41

Inexpensive Prevention Becomes Expensive Treatment

Wen a nutritional product has powerful effects, pharmaceutical manufacturers may change its chemical structure slightly in order to obtain a patent. Companies know how to do this, because many—if not most—drugs are mimics of natural substances. Naturally occurring products are modified not only to get patents but also to make drugs that are better absorbed, stay in the body longer, or degrade more slowly on the pharmacy shelf.

Fish oil has long been a nutritional supplement; many older people remember their grandmothers dosing them with cod liver oil when they were young. The omega-3 fatty acids in fish oil are beneficial in a number of conditions related to inflammation, including America's number one killer: heart attacks (Silletta, Pioggiarella, Levantesi, et al. 2009, 440–47; Gruppo Italiano 1999, 447–55; O'Keefe & Harris 2000, 607–14).

Glaxo and Amarin wanted to bring fish oil and its health benefits to the pharmaceutical marketplace, so each company modified the omega-3 fatty acids somewhat differently by adding an extra chemical group, called an ester, to them. When the body takes the ester group off, the omega-3 fatty acids are released. Those modified omega-3 fatty acids, called "pro-drugs" because they turn into active drugs in the body, were patentable. The two manufacturers could put their fatty acid esters

(Lovaza and Vascepa, respectively) through the FDA's approval process and come out with two distinct fish oil–based drugs. Both products are approved for lowering excessively high triglycerides, a fatty substance in the blood that predisposes a person to heart disease.

Only those two manufacturers can now legally go to doctors and tell them about the cardiovascular benefits of their products. If a nutritional supplement maker or a national pharmacy chain selling fish oil told physicians about the same benefits, it could be prosecuted and sent to prison because the products haven't received the FDA's formal approval to treat cardiovascular disease.

Doctors get most of their information about new products from pharmaceutical reps. The makers of Lovaza and Vascepa tell physicians that their fish oil products are the only ones that are good enough to be approved by the FDA. They are not likely to tell doctors that their patients can purchase the active ingredient of these pro-drugs without a prescription at a much lower price.

My sister asked her doctor about prescription fish oil because she had been taking it as a nutritional supplement. Even though she had a good health insurance policy, her co-pay for Lovaza would have been comparable to what she was already paying for her over-the-counter product. Naturally, her insurance company would pick up most of the bill. When Lovaza first came out, it was 8–9 times as expensive as a comparable dose of high-quality fish oil (Faloon 2011, 204).

Insurance companies won't pay the small cost of high-quality, over-the-counter fish oil, but they will pay for the high-priced prescription pro-drugs of the active ingredient because those products are FDA-approved. In the long run, paying more than we need to for a supplement or drug means a lower standard of care for us all.

Like many fish oil products, Lovaza contains significant amounts (5.3 ppb) of polychlorinated biphenyls (PCBs). Although some highly refined over-the-counter products contain less (e.g., OmegaRx has 0.8 ppb) (MacFarlane n.d.), vendors can't legally market their product to doctors as a more purified version of the fish oil "drug" without jumping through the FDA's regulatory hoops.

Age-related macular degeneration (AMD), the leading cause of blindness in the elderly, has no effective drug treatment. One study with daily high-dose fish oil (OmegaRx), providing 3.4 grams of eicosapentaenoic acid (EPA) and 1.6 grams of docosahexaenoic acid (DHA), partially reversed AMD after 6 months. All 25 patients showed improvement in their vision (Georgiou, Neokleous, Nicolaou, et al. 2014, 8–11; Georgiou & Prokopiou 2015, 205–15). Lower doses of EPA (0.65–0.85 grams) had no effect, even when DHA was higher (2.5 grams per day) (Gerstenblith, Baskin, Shah, et al. 2013, 365–69; AREDS2 2013, 2005–15).

Because blindness is so debilitating and because fish oil has few side effects, doctors would likely recommend it to their elderly patients if they knew about its benefits. However, sellers of prescription fish oil and over-the-counter products could be prosecuted by the FDA for visiting doctors to educate them about those benefits without going through years of Amendment-driven studies. Thankfully, researchers can inform physicians at conferences by presenting their findings, but most doctors are too busy to attend those meetings. Consequently, medical practice is often years—if not decades—behind cutting-edge research.

Chapter 42

New Dietary Ingredients Regulations Thwart Prevention

I n 1994, Congress considered several bills to give the FDA more power over nutritional supplement manufacturing and labeling. Consumer and supplement manufacturers were appalled and lobbied heavily for more of a hands-off policy. In response to this outcry, Congress passed the Dietary Supplement Health and Education Act of 1994 (DSHEA) instead and designated dietary supplements as food, not drugs.

The FDA decided that DSHEA applied only to products that could be documented with invoices, catalogs, or other written items before 1994. If a compound was marketed for a short time, such items might no longer be available. Sworn statements or affidavits from those involved in pre-1994 marketing were deemed inadequate by the FDA. The exact form of the nutrient must have been marketed as a stand-alone supplement, not in a combination product (Arhangelsky 2011).

In addition, the FDA claims that a supplement is not grandfathered in under DSHEA if a drug company has ever submitted an IND for it. In 2005, Biostratum Inc. asked the FDA to prohibit the sale of dietary supplements containing pyridoxamine dihydrochloride, which is a naturally occurring form of vitamin B6 present in fish, milk, and other foods. Biostratum argued that those supplements were unlawful because the company had filed an IND with the FDA in 1999 to alleviate or prevent kidney disease in diabetics. In 2009, the FDA agreed that any compound, even a naturally occurring substance, was a drug instead of a supplement if an IND had been filed (Kennedy 2013).

Biostratum, like many smaller companies, found it difficult to raise money for its Phase 3 trials. NephroGenex Inc. acquired Pyridorin®, the trade name for pyridoxamine dihydrocholoride, and also appears to be having trouble funding the Phase 3 studies (StreetInsider.com. 2016). Meanwhile, US diabetics and their doctors probably don't realize that they might be able to avoid kidney failure by taking this natural product. Even if they are aware, this supplement cannot be legally sold in the United States because it is under development as a drug. Before the Amendments, this natural form of vitamin B6 would not have been removed from the market.

The regulatory fallout from the Amendments is depriving American diabetics of the chance to save or delay the kidney deterioration that their disease causes. Indeed, this vitamin might protect the kidney in other patients as well, but the Amendments have condemned those people to an early death because the FDA has deemed pyridoxamine dihydrocholoride a drug.

Twenty years ago, FDA could not act to take a dietary supplement off the market unless it could prove that the supplement presented a significant or unreasonable risk of illness or injury.... Today, FDA can take any dietary supplement or category of supplements off the market if the FDA summarily concludes there to be a potential to cause injury [including–based on the fact that the supplement (as in all things ingestible)—could cause injury at some dose level]; it was made by a company that did not satisfy GMP record-keeping requirements; or it is a supplement that FDA believes could possibly cause injury to some segment of the population (e.g., again as in all things ingestible, it may cause an allergic reaction). There is in this no need to prove any finished product injurious and no limit to government power; it is unbridled discretion. It means that no one who makes or distributes a dietary supplement can rest assured that a safe product is free from summary removal from the market by the FDA, according to that agency's whim or caprice.

—Jonathan Emord, lead counsel in several landmark cases against the FDA,
January 2013

If a company has a truly new dietary ingredient that it wants to market, it must submit a 75-day premarket notification to the FDA. In 2011, the proposed notification took an estimated 100–250 hours to prepare. Dr. Joanna Shepherd Bailey, Emory University Professor of Law and Economics, estimates the animal and human product safety studies that the FDA wanted for a new dietary ingredients (NDI) notification would require $450,000 to $6.6 million per NDI notification (US FDA 2011). Such costs would have a chilling effect on the supplement industry.

Some people believe that the FDA doesn't regulate supplements, but that is not the case. The FDA establishes Good Manufacturing Rules (GMPs) for them, courtesy of DSHEA. Just as with drugs, failure to keep good GMP records can result in withdrawal of the product from the market.

Chapter 43

Thalidomide Takes Us Back to the Future

n the summer of 1998, the FDA quietly approved thalidomide for prevention and treatment of the skin lesions of leprosy (US FDA 1998). The reviled drug that spawned the deadly Amendments turned out to alleviate some of the problems caused by this dread disease.

In May 2006, the FDA approved thalidomide for a rare cancer, multiple myeloma. Thalidomide prevents angiogenesis, the process by which tumors increase their blood supply and metastasize. Consequently, studies in other cancers are ongoing. Thalidomide also modulates the immune system, making it a potentially useful drug for transplantation, HIV-related Kaposi's sarcoma (a skin cancer), and inflammatory disease (see US FDA n.d.a. for a list of ongoing testing for thalidomide in the United States).

In a sense, we've come full circle. Thalidomide, a sleeping drug that was safer than barbiturates, was intended to save lives. Perhaps in other life-threatening diseases, it still will. The same drug that kills or maims the developing baby might very well save its parents from death by disease, possibly by the same mechanism of action.

Prostaglandin E_1 (PGE1) is another such drug. Made in every cell of the body, PGE1 is part of the eicosanoid pathway, which is tweaked by aspirin, fish oil, and other anti-inflammatory compounds. Upjohn developed this natural product in order to keep a critical blood vessel, known as the ductus arteriosus, open in babies awaiting surgery for heart defects. Should the ductus close as it normally does after birth, those infants would not get enough oxygen to survive. They were known as "blue babies" because their healthy pink tint turned blue when their red blood cells were rapidly depleted of their life-giving oxygen. By keeping the ductus opened, PGE1 allowed the babies to stabilize and go into heart surgery with the best chance for survival.

Alprostadil (PGE_1) infusion could save three out of four such infants (Atik, Gutierrez, Filho, et al. 1989, 93–97). The Upjohn Company developed PGE_1 to save those babies even though it could not sell enough of this compound to recover its costs. Upjohn executives felt that saving the lives of infants was the best advertisement for its anticipated line of new prostaglandin products.

PGE_1 is also one of the natural hormones involved in labor induction. Therefore, women who did not go into labor when expected were sometimes given PGE_1 instead of a C-section or caesarean. Eventually, physicians began using PGE_1 to induce "delivery" of an unwanted fetus in the first 3 months of pregnancy instead of surgically aborting it. Ironically, anti-abortion activists called for a ban on PGE_1, unaware that this drug was first marketed—at a loss—to save babies' lives.

In still another ironic twist of fate, PGE_1 sales started to soar many years after its introduction, even though there were not enough blue babies or abortions to account for them. Upjohn discovered that men were getting PGE_1 from their pharmacist and injecting it into their male member to alleviate their erectile dysfunction. In the late 1980s, this widespread concern was not talked about much. PGE_1 is currently available for this indication, but the market leader is the well-known Viagra.

Both thalidomide and PGE_1 have saved lives and taken them. The drug that saves the life of one person may very well kill another. Drugs are powerful substances and must be used at the right dose, at the right time, for the right conditions.

Chapter 44

How the Amendments Have Institutionalized Corruption

Most critics of the pharmaceutical companies are unaware of how the Amendments are still reshaping the drug companies, the FDA, and the supplement industry, while shifting our medical paradigm from prevention to treatment. Because they don't understand how the current regulatory climate affects what drug companies do, they've simply assumed that the pharmaceutical industry suffers more greed than other industries.

Everyone wants the best for themselves; this greed is built into our genes as a survival mechanism. One person's greed, however, can actually serve another person's need. In theory at least, this is how the marketplace works: you make a drug that will save my life, and I buy it from you, delighted that it exists. You make a profit for your effort, and I stay alive because of it. It's a win–win scenario.

As we've seen, the Amendments have greatly distorted this simple, straightforward arrangement. By imposing ever-increasing manufacturing, advertising, and development restrictions, the Amendments squelched small, efficient drug companies, thereby creating a pharmaceutical cartel. The same regulatory process that creates the pharmaceutical cartel also shifts resources from research to development and from prevention to treatment. As a result, we become sicker as the innovations that might have saved us are lost.

The regulations that create this cartel penalize honesty and fair play, while rewarding guile and deception. The courts ruled that drug companies would have no recourse if the FDA denied an approval for the most trivial of reasons or dragged out its review so that a competitor—in which the regulator might have a hidden financial interest—could be first to market. The Amendments, as well as the court decisions surrounding them, gave the FDA the power to make or break a drug company as the agency pleased and with minimal blowback.

Power corrupts. In the few instances where the courts ruled against the FDA, the agency simply ignored court orders. With almost unlimited resources from our tax dollars to appeal unfavorable decisions, the FDA could expect to eventually have those rulings reversed.

Even with all of the power that FDA regulators have to make or break drug companies with few, if any, consequences, the Amendments have put the regulators at risk as well. Every drug is a land mine for FDA regulators, because every drug has side effects that threaten the public's belief that FDA approval means safety. When harmful side effects come to light and when people complain to their representatives, the regulators are chastised publically and angrily by Congress on national television.

When the FDA denies a drug approval, patients who pinned their hopes on that drug revile the agency on the Internet and on social media. The regulators are in a no-win situation. They're damned if they do approve novel drugs and damned if they don't.

On the pharmaceutical side of the equation, drug companies have often felt victimized by an FDA so empowered by the Amendments. Small companies felt that they were treated unfairly when they didn't have adequate time to upgrade their manufacturing facilities to the new GMP standards. Firms that sold combination antibiotics were frustrated because they were not allowed to face their accusers and openly present their case. Instead of receiving time and guidance to upgrade their facilities or do the studies required by the Amendments, the firms were deprived of substantial income or went bankrupt. The industry's expectation of due process was undermined. This atmosphere sets the stage for fighting fire with fire or responding in ways that could be considered unethical.

Because the FDA doesn't actually have an objective way to balance the potential benefits and risks of a new drug when considering an approval, a company's survival doesn't necessarily depend on its ability to make drugs that save lives, relieve pain, or make our lives better. Companies must do whatever it takes to keep on the regulators' good side; simply having drugs that are reasonably safe and effective is not necessarily enough.

Consequently, some firms may take the back door to approvals, opting to stroke the egos of the regulators, to co-opt, or even to bribe them (Chapter 4). In an environment where fair play has already been undermined by the courts, thereby giving regulators life-and-death power over a company's survival, such unscrupulous tactics are less likely to seem illegitimate and are more likely to seem a necessary way to do business. The primary focus shifts from saving lives to placating the regulators. Discovering new drugs takes second place to managing the regulatory red tape. Without the regulators in your corner, helping the sick and dying becomes nearly impossible.

Both the agency and the drug companies will experience more corruption when approvals are based on politics rather than on science. In such an environment, survival might seem to depend on resorting to unsavory and unethical tactics.

Chapter 45

The Amendments Are a Cure Worse than the "Disease"

B y continuing to reshape the pharmaceutical industry, the regulatory climate, and the supplement or natural product industry in a way that shifts our health care paradigm from prevention to treatment, the Amendments have stopped us from realizing the Golden Age of Health that should have already been ours. Instead, half of the Americans who have died since passage of the Amendments have done so prematurely. Because this estimate is a conservative one, the stark reality is that each one of us—whether we are regulators, drug company employees, doctors, patients, or part of the public—has likely lost years of our lives because of the legislation. Moveover, our quality of life has been compromised as well.

Many Americans died waiting for lifesaving drugs because the Amendments tripled development time. Those wealthy enough will sometimes go overseas where drugs can make it through the regulatory red tape faster. Still others take matters into their own hands and obtain unapproved drugs in the black market, thus risking prosecution and incarceration for trying to stay alive. Terminally ill Americans were told by the courts that they had no constitutional right to save their lives if it meant taking drugs that did not have FDA approval. As a result, desperate patients still try to manufacture promising new drugs in their own kitchens. An estimated 15 million Americans have lost their lives as a result of Amendment-driven delays in getting new drugs to market.

When new drugs are in the regulatory pipeline, patients can at least become aware of them and seek them elsewhere. The 50% of drugs in clinical testing that are not deemed economically feasible might still be visible to those seeking out a lifesaving drug for their disease. However, when innovative new products die on the pharmaceutical manufacturers' shelves before they even enter clinical testing, very few people know about their potential. Conservative estimates suggest that about 26.7 million Americans have lost their lives because innovations that would have been economically feasible before the Amendments would drive a company into bankruptcy today.

We've paid for the Amendments, not just in lives, but with our hard-earned money as well. Our pharmacy bills are as much as 40 times more for new drugs than they would be in the absence of the Amendments. Because drug prices are driven by ever-increasing development costs, they will continue to rise if we don't intervene.

We might be willing to put up with delays and soaring pharmaceutical prices—as costly as they are in terms of lives and money—if the drugs on our pharmacy shelves were safer than they were before 1962. By every measure considered, however, post-Amendment drugs appear to be no safer than pre-Amendment ones. If anything, the evidence suggests that the Amendments made drugs less safe. This finding only confirms what many already knew in 1962: we don't know enough to be able to predict every side effect. Some will be seen only after large numbers of people have taken a drug.

By making development so costly, the Amendments have changed the kind of drugs that manufacturers take to market. Before 1962, most drugs were taken for a relatively short time. Today, most drugs are intended to be used for years or even decades so that development costs can be recovered. Even so, only 2–3 drugs out of 10 do so; the solvency of most pharmaceutical firms depends on having an occasional blockbuster drug to offset the much more frequent losers.

Because pharmaceuticals are often taken for a lifetime, our bodies become depleted of critical nutrients used in drug detoxification. An increasing number of people are taking more than a dozen drugs daily, so the body has to work harder, thereby depleting even more nutrients.

Mixing drugs can be deadly because the drugs can interact in unexpected ways. Consequently, properly prescribed drugs have become a leading cause of death in recent years, especially as the number of drugs that each person takes has risen. The Amendments, which were designed to keep us safe, have almost guaranteed us deadly side effects.

Because of the increasing risk, cost, and time involved in taking a new drug to market, investors demand a greater return on their investment. Drug company profits are, to a large extent, a reflection of how risky and uncertain that drug development has become. If profits fall, investors put their money in safer ventures, and new drug development is curtailed accordingly. Because critics of the pharmaceutical companies are largely unaware of how the Amendments have increased the risk of trying to develop a new drug, they erroneously interpret investors' demands for a higher return as greed on the part of the drug companies.

The FDA has been given the power, through the Amendments, to determine which companies will prosper. By demanding more studies of one firm than another or simply by dragging their feet, regulators can manipulate the industry, and the courts have virtually given the regulators carte blanche.

In such an atmosphere, where approvals and company survival can turn on the whim of a regulator, corruption at both the FDA and the pharmaceutical industry is rewarded. The Amendments set the stage for the passage of PDUFA. Unfortunately, PDUFA creates a severe conflict of interest for regulators by supplying more than 70% of the salaries for those who evaluate new drugs.

Because a delayed approval can mean bankruptcy, especially for a small company, the pharmaceutical industry has been consolidating for the past several decades. Unless drug development costs stop rising, this trend will continue until the current pharmaceutical cartel becomes a duopoly or monopoly.

As regulations become more demanding, older drugs become less profitable. The companies that originally developed those agents or marketed the generic version eventually find the older drugs to be less profitable than newer drugs. One by one, pharmaceutical firms stop manufacturing the older drugs until only one supplier is left. Small firms looking for windfall profits buy the rights from the lone supplier and hike prices, secure in the knowledge that any generic competitor will have to wade through at least 3 years of FDA-mandated regulatory red tape before reaching the market. Unbridled greed is rewarded, courtesy of the Amendments and their aftermath.

The continuing increase in development costs that drive the consolidation of the drug companies also shifts money from research to development, thereby ensuring that innovation will be stymied even more than it is now. Less innovation means drugs that could have improved the quality of our lives and given us more longevity will never make it to our pharmacy shelves.

Stem cells are one of the most-promising areas of innovation today, but the research in this area is being driven offshore by an FDA empowered by the Amendments and courts. Most stem cell procedures concentrate a patient's own cells from fat or bone marrow and return the cells in concentrated form to the area of the body that needs repair or rejuvenation. The FDA believes that such cells—your cells—are a drug that the agency should control. Consequently, unless you are wealthy enough to go offshore, you can't get the most cutting-edge therapy.

If you are a physician and have a novel cancer treatment, you'll find that the FDA isn't fond of single investigators. The regulators want new drug developers to have deep pockets so they can get enough studies done to show their due diligence if side effects come to the attention of Congress.

Because almost half of their salaries are funded through PDUFA, regulators want to protect drug companies. If supplement manufacturers can tell people about the lifesaving benefits of their products or how the natural products might improve their quality of life, the drug industry may suffer. Regulators might be let go as a result. Consequently, the FDA works against food producers and supplement manufacturers who try to share the health benefits of their products with consumers.

The New Dietary Ingredients regulations will ensure that the best of tomorrow's new nutrients will become expensive treatments instead of being marketed as inexpensive prevention. When the compounds are chosen to be developed as drugs, they will be pulled from (or never enter) the market. Instead of quick access to inexpensive, lifesaving nutrients, we will all be forced to wait until the products successfully navigate the ever-increasing regulatory red tape and become expensive drugs.

The ongoing shift from prevention to treatment is probably more deadly than the negative impact of the Amendments on the drug industry. All of us have probably lost additional years of our lives or had the quality of our lives compromised because of the censorship of information about inexpensive nutritional substances. Educating doctors is essentially illegal without going through the FDA regulatory red tape. The shift from prevention to treatment, with its added medical costs, has deprived us of both health and wealth.

For example, the American thalidomide incident, more horrific than the European one, was a direct result of the censorship imposed by the 1962 Amendments on a single vitamin (folic acid) for one simple use (preventing certain types of birth defects). Doubling vitamin D levels may be able to add 2 years to the average person's life, but the Amendments forbid manufacturers from sharing this information with doctors. Similarly, up to 96,000 people a year die from omega-3 deficiency (Danaei, Ding, Mozaffarian, et al. 2009, e1000058), but even the sellers of prescription fish oil can't point this out to doctors because the only indication for their fish oil "drugs" is lowering triglycerides. Ironically, the public often learns about preventative practices on the Internet and must often educate their physicians on such subjects rather than vice versa.

Our doctors are, for the most part, unaware that many chronic conditions can be controlled, prevented, or largely alleviated with nutritional supplements or foods or both. They continuously add more drugs to our daily regimen, because although the drug reps can legally educate the doctors, supplement manufacturers generally cannot. Overworked doctors, whose numbers are limited by state regulations (Ruwart 2015, 67–82), rarely have time to review drug information on the Internet, let alone learn about vitamins and how their optimization enhances health.

Indeed, doctors are often not even aware of many off-label uses of approved drugs, because the information that drug reps can convey is limited as well. For example, because of the Amendments, most doctors were unaware of aspirin's protection of the heart for almost two decades. That ignorance cost the American public an estimated 1.7 million lives.

Through an incremental process, the FDA has been able to put itself in a position where the agency can arbitrarily take any supplement off the market (Emord 2013). Not enough information is currently available to give a reasonable estimate of how many Americans have died, because the Amendments have made it difficult for sellers of vitamins and nutrients to educate doctors about the benefits of their products. Most likely, we have all been affected.

The most conservative estimate would be to assume that many of the lost pharmaceutical innovations would have been nutritional supplements that the drug industry would have been able to offer the public without having to go through the arduous regulatory pathway created by the Amendments. In other words, in the most conservative estimate, the one out of four Americans who died prematurely would have included those who died from lack of prevention. However, the more likely scenario is that we have all lost years of our lives to the Amendments.

Regulations are just as powerful as drugs are, with the potential to have life-threatening side effects, even beyond our own borders. What happened in the United States has rippled outward into the world, resulting in millions more premature deaths. Because most innovation happens in the United States, its attenuation by the Amendments meant that other nations were denied lifesaving drugs too. The research, as well as the knowledge that would have come from new discoveries, was also lost. In addition, disease prevention was thwarted by the FDA's insistence (and the courts' agreement) that making a claim that a nutrient could atten-uate or alleviate disease changed that nutrient into a drug. The Golden Age of Health that humankind might have enjoyed was thus thwarted by the Amendments.

Chapter 46

We Are All Hamed by the Amendments

The Amendments have deprived all of us—regulators, doctors, drug industry scientists, and executives, as well as the public—of new, innovative therapies, while greatly delaying those we do get. Instead of emphasizing prevention, most of our remaining innovations are aimed at treatment. Consequently, instead of living a long and healthy life, many of us die prematurely.

Regulators might feel empowered by the Amendments. Pharmaceutical managers may be secretly heartened when their smaller competitors are destroyed or forced to merge because of the regulatory pressure. However, the ultimate price that they pay for the temporary advantages afforded by the Amendments is a shorter life for themselves and their loved ones. No matter how much power or wealth a person has, he or she cannot buy a lifesaving innovation that is unavailable because of the Amendments.

Dr. Richard Pazdur, head of the oncology section of the FDA, learned this lesson the hard way. Pazdur would not approve new cancer drugs unless they lengthened the lives of patients. Such studies take many years to complete; this requirement slowed down the approval of new cancer drugs and brought criticism from patient advocacy groups such as the Abigail Alliance (Harris 2009). However, his attitude changed when his wife was diagnosed with ovarian cancer and eventually lost her 3-year battle against it. Working with her to get access to drugs still in the regulatory pipeline helped him realize just how deadly that regulatory delays are.

Following his wife's death in November 2015, Pazdur has, in his own words, "been on a jihad to streamline the review process and get things out the door faster." Review time for cancer drugs has gone from 6 months to 5 months. Although applauded by some, Pazdur was criticized as becoming too soft on the drug companies, recklessly approving drugs without adequate consideration (Harris 2016). As usual, regulators are in a no-win situation: they are criticized by one group when they delay approvals and criticized by another when they accelerate approvals.

Although shortening the review process by a month will save lives, the real problem—more than a decade of FDA-mandated studies—remains. Since 1962, what is expected of drug companies has incrementally increased; the regulatory burden continues to grow. Because the development process has been institutionalized over time, no one person at the agency can change it.

An FDA commissioner who tried to eliminate or streamline part of the process so that drugs could get to market earlier would enrage those who erroneously equate long development times with safety. Indeed, FDA Commissioner Frank Young felt driven to leave the agency in 1989, in part, because he allowed AIDS patients to bring small quantities of drugs that had been approved overseas into the United States for their personal use. Instead of being recognized as a gesture of compassion, Young's action was thought by many to be irresponsible.

All of us are at risk when regulations are so strict that we lose more than half of our innovations—and must wait a decade or more for the ones we do get. All of us are at risk when manufacturers, who know their products best, can't share lifesaving information with our health care providers. All of us are at risk when our prevention options are artificially limited by the Amendment-driven regulations.

Chapter 47

What Would We Have Had without the Amendments?

W hat would our health care landscape look like if the Amendments had never been passed? Although it is impossible to say for certain, given the trends in the 1960s and 1970s, it's likely that prevention would have become the predominant medical paradigm, a development that would have likely added many years to each of our lives.

Drug companies would likely have remained engaged in this modality, because they would have been able to make health claims for their products without running afoul of the FDA or risking delays of their next NCE approval. Some companies did impressive research on natural products before the Amendments made this work unsustainable.

Consequently, pharmaceutical innovation would likely have included vitamins, minerals, and other natural substances, which could have been marketed profitably for disease prevention and treatment. Without the FDA's bias against combinations drugs, supplements could be added to pharmaceuticals to avoid the depletion of nutrients that occur during detoxification. Indeed, such combination products might have saved us from many of the deadly side effects of powerful pharmaceuticals or kept products such as Vioxx from ever reaching the market (Chapter 32).

Innovations would come to market more quickly. Because manufacturers have great incentive to be first to market, the pre-Amendment development timeline of 4 years might have been shortened further without
compromising safety. AIDS patients might not have had to rely on the
black market for their drugs, and cancer patients would have had earlier
access to new therapies, which might have also been less toxic.

Nutritional products for prevention and treatment of disease would
have been more thoroughly investigated. If pharmaceutical firms didn't
have to pay the high costs of development that they do today, they'd have
more than three times as much money for research. If companies could
market supplements that were safe for the intended use, which is the
pre-Amendment standard, some of that research would have likely involved natural products.

Without the soaring costs of regulatory red tape, drug companies could
profitably develop drugs for short-term usage or a small patient base. The
Orphan Drug Act, which creates monopolies and the astronomical prices
associated with lack of competition, would never have been passed.

Without the Amendments, small companies would not have been
driven out of business. They would have continued to compete with the
larger firms. With more products to choose from, including more alternatives to branded drugs, our pharmacy bills would likely be less than
10%—and possibly as low as 2.5%—of what they now are. Competition
keeps prices low, while regulation drives them up.

> *... what's needed is more competition. Warts and all, the competitive
> marketplace is the best protector of consumers.*
> —Murray Weidenbaum, Professor and Honorary Chairman of the Murray Weidenbaum
> Center on the Economy, Government, and Public Policy at Washington University

Without pharmaceutical cartels, as well as FDA approval as the gold
standard of quality, a firm's brand name would have continued to be crucial to a company's success. The marketplace would likely have capped
consumer waste at 10–20%, as it did before passage of the Amendments.

Compared to the greater than 1,000% markup created by the Amendments, the American public would enjoy considerable savings.

If such a scenario seems too good to be true, consider the evolution of surgical practice in the United States. Doctors didn't need to go through the FDA or any involved regulatory process to develop transplantation, knee and hip replacements, cardiac bypass, reconnection of a severed finger, or lifesaving trauma techniques. The United States has the best surgeons in the world; doctors come here from all over the world to train.

The ability of our surgeons to experiment has its downside too. Cardiac bypass was overused; many patients underwent unnecessary procedures. Studies finally determined who benefited from the surgery and who did not. During the evolution of medicine, such overtreatment will inevitably happen.

Slowing down the introduction of a lifesaving technique until it can be well defined, however, results in an even greater loss of life. This is a high price to pay for medical certainty, especially if it's *your* life. Allowing those who wish to try something new, with its attendant risks, gives valuable information that promotes progress. Those who want to play it safe and wait until the innovation proves itself should be able to do that too. That's the freedom on which our nation was founded.

We've already seen how this freedom plays out in the supplement industry. Some people consider such products worthless and don't take them. Some people believe that their lives are saved or made better by them. Because we all have different genetics and environments, supplements are likely to help some and not others. We each make a choice and live with the consequences.

Because supplements are not as highly regulated as prescription drugs, their prices are much lower than today's pharmaceuticals, unless they are put through the regulatory process—as fish oil was. In general, they are also less likely to cause deadly side effects because our bodies recognize them and know how to handle them. However, some people will still react negatively to them because of our biological diversity. Even something that is good for most may not be good for all.

Chapter 48

Where Did the Amendments Go Wrong

hether we are regulators, pharmaceutical employees, doctors, or patients, we all are—first and foremost—human beings. About 90% of us will die from disease. If we want to live longer, healthier lives without a financial outlay for new drugs that will drive us into bankruptcy, we need to fix the problems created by the Amendments. Like a cancer, the problems get worse every year as the regulations metastasize throughout the drug, medical, nutritional, and preventative health industries.

The Amendments were not just regulatory overkill; they were actually unnecessary. Thalidomide was never approved in the United States because the regulations in place in the early 1960s had already given the FDA enough power to stop drugs that looked as if they might have safety problems.

Because some critics of the drug companies don't understand the role of the Amendments in harming the American public, they want to fix things with more regulations instead of getting rid of the ones that caused problems in the first place. Many people cling to the idea that because the *intention* of the regulations was to protect the consumer, they must surely do so. Nothing could be further from the truth. Regulations are just as powerful as drugs are and can have side effects that are just as deadly.

Although beyond the scope of this book, the discovery that regulations harm the very people they are intended to help is not new. Indeed, regulations generally create cartels that decrease competition, increase the price of the product or service, decrease the amount of quality service delivered, and undercut lifesaving and cost-cutting innovation. Consequently, states with the most-stringent regulations for optometrists have the most blindness, and those with the most-stringent regulations for electricians have the most accidental electrocutions (Carroll & Gaston 1981, 959–76; Carroll & Gaston 1983, 139–46). When regulations price the poor out of the marketplace, they don't visit the eye doctor or call an electrician. Consequently, they often lose their sight or even their lives.

Likewise, the poor or those on fixed incomes, such as the elderly, can't afford the high prices of their medicine—courtesy of the Amendments. Consequently, they do without and pay with more suffering, or worse, with their lives.

To fix the issues caused by the Amendments, we need to understand why the regulations have failed us so we don't repeat our mistakes. Why didn't the Amendments give us safer, more low-cost, and effective drugs? In addition to the regulatory impact on the cost and quantity of quality service delivered, the regulators, unlike the American public and health care professionals, rarely are directly harmed by their decisions.

For example, when regulators prevent patients from buying a new, promising drug that has not yet been approved, the patients—not the regulators—suffer the consequences. The regulators might be criticized for foot-dragging, but they can't be sued for withholding treatment. A doctor who doesn't prescribe an appropriate, FDA-approved drug to a patient, conversely, can be sued for malpractice, perhaps even manslaughter if the patient dies (Barcus 2010). In contrast, regulators have no legal responsibility if people die because the FDA keeps a lifesaving drug from terminally ill patients.

If regulators do approve a drug and if it has horrific side effects, Congress will hold hearings and publicly criticize the FDA. Because every drug has side effects, regulators are hesitant to approve a new drug unless they have a literal truckload of studies to prove their due diligence. When they make a mistake and a drug must be withdrawn, the drug companies—not the regulators—will be sued for damages, even if tens of thousands of people die from that drug's side effects.

Because regulators are not legally liable if they withhold lifesaving drugs from the market or if they approve deadly drugs, their incentives are skewed. They need not fear legal action; their access to taxpayer dollars means that they can keep appealing court decisions until they get their desired outcome. Instead, regulators focus on avoiding the wrath of those who pay their salaries: Congress and the drug companies. Consequently, regulators often ignore the needs of the very people they are supposed to be helping—the American public.

As a result, each of us likely has had our lives shortened by the Amendments. We have lost access to the Golden Age of Health that we should have otherwise enjoyed.

Chapter 49

How Do We Fix the Problems Caused by the Amendments?

The biggest problem with most regulation, the Amendments included, is that the decision making is in the hands of regulators who don't suffer the consequences of their decisions. The solution is not to make regulators legally liable but to put the final choice in the hands of those who must experience the consequences. Because patients will live or die by this decision, they must be the ones to make it, hopefully with the advice of trusted health professionals.

One way to ensure that consumers, not bureaucrats, have the final say in what drugs patients can take would be to dismantle the FDA. However, the FDA regulates not only pharmaceuticals but also foods, veterinary products, medical devices and radiological equipment, nutritional products, and tobacco. Because this book makes the case only that the Amendments were regulatory overkill in their reshaping of the pharmaceutical, medical, and nutraceutical industries, the suggested remedies will be limited to undoing the damage caused by those Amendments. In allowing us finally to reclaim the Golden Age of Health that should be ours, the success of such remedies sets the stage for further deregulation.

Specifically, the recommended remedies are as follows:

1. Repeal the 1962 Amendments.

2. Revoke the FDA's ability to approve new drugs. Instead, allow the
    FDA to make reviews, recommendations, or certifications.
3. Pass the Health Freedom Act HR 2117 or similar legislation to nullify
    the court decision that making a health claim for a food or nutrient
    makes it a drug.

Together, those three changes would allow us to claim our lost Golden
Age of Health.

REPEAL THE 1962 AMENDMENTS

The Amendments were clearly regulatory overkill. They were not needed
to prevent the thalidomide tragedy, which was thwarted in the United States
by the regulations already in place. Instead, they delayed the entry of lifesaving drugs into the market, destroyed 50–80% of our pharmaceutical
innovations, increased drug prices by 10–40 fold, and censored lifesaving
information about vitamins and other natural products. In the process, the
Amendments created an American thalidomide instead of preventing one
and have, in all likelihood, shortened the lives of virtually every American.

Ironically, we have no evidence at all that the Amendments have kept
dangerous drugs off the market. Indeed, Vioxx, the biggest drug disaster
of all time, may actually have been caused by the distorted incentives
created by the Amendments.

REVOKE THE FDA'S ABILITY TO APPROVE NEW DRUGS

To many people, letting patients buy drugs that they want at any
stage of the approval process will seem like a drastic and dangerous solution. Couldn't we simply do away with the Amendments and go back to
the days before they were passed? Probably not: between 1962 and the
present, the courts have consistently ruled that drug companies cannot

sue the FDA if the agency withdraws a drug from the market or fails to approve it in the first place. Courts have also ruled that when a manufacturer makes a health claim for a food or supplement, that product becomes a drug and is subject to FDA's regulations. Doing away with the Amendments wouldn't change those critical rulings.

Consequently, the FDA could demand the same studies that it did under the Amendments, and the drug companies would have little recourse if they wanted their products approved. When the FDA demanded expensive and time-consuming effectiveness studies, pharmaceutical firms might sue on the grounds that the studies were no longer required for approval. However, the FDA could easily argue that the required studies were needed primarily to make sure the drug was safe in larger populations. Getting effectiveness data would be designated as a secondary consideration but a seemingly reasonable one, given that the long and involved study must be done anyway for a stepped-up, newly defined version of safety.

Courts would be unlikely to side with the drug companies against another government agency, especially because it would seem prudent to demand longer, more involved studies in the false belief that they will ensure more safety. Even if courts ruled against the agency, the FDA would likely ignore the ruling as it has done in the past. The firm that brought court action would likely find that the FDA would demand more studies from the whistleblower than from their competitors. A company that challenged the FDA could—and probably would—be put out of business with the additional costs. Consequently, any solution that doesn't allow drugs to be marketed without FDA approval will be doomed to failure.

Wouldn't some patients make bad drug choices? Of course they would, just as the FDA has made some bad choices in drug approvals. Our science is just not good enough to prevent some bad outcomes, no matter who the decision maker is. Total safety is not possible. To the extent that we still don't understand how the body works—and that means to a great extent—we are all guinea pigs taking drugs and nutritional products that may or may not be suitable for us. The best we can hope to do—whether we are patients, doctors, or regulators—is make an *informed* decision.

Having *all* of the available information is the very definition of "informed." I currently chair an IRB (Institutional Review Board) that vets the informed consent that drug companies must give human subjects undergoing new drug testing. The IRB must make sure that each person gets full disclosure about both potential risks and benefits. If this information is not provided, the study is considered unethical and cannot be legally undertaken.

To the extent that the FDA prohibits what patients and doctors can be told about any therapy or supplement, making an informed decision isn't possible. The FDA's unethical restrictions on free speech must also end so that informed decision making can occur. A health claim, such as "these studies suggest that this drug (or nutrient) might be useful in Disease X," shouldn't have to be vetted by the FDA's regulatory process. A disclaimer, such as "These statements have not been evaluated by the Food and Drug Administration," could alert consumers that the FDA has not signed off on those claims.

Because patients must experience the consequences of any medical decision, they should ultimately be the ones to make it. They should be able to purchase innovative drugs at any stage of development, and drug companies should be able to legally supply them.

In a very real sense, patients make such decisions today. Their doctors explain to them what their different options are, but patients ultimately decide whether or not to take the recommended drugs or treatments. The only difference is that more drugs at earlier stages of development would also be available.

For decades, patients have wanted this option and have been willing to accept the risks that such a choice might entail. As early as the 1980s, life-extension researchers Durk Pearson and Sandy Shaw suggested a split-label approach to supplements that would give both manufacturers and the FDA equal space to share information with the consumer (Pearson & Shaw 1993, 7). Shortly thereafter, the AIDS community simply ignored the FDA's regulations; today, some ALS patients and others with limited options are making unapproved drugs in their kitchens. The Abigail Alliance and terminally ill cancer patients sued the FDA unsuccessfully to legalize their access to unapproved drugs so they would not have to break the law. Some patients, notably those with ALS, still try to concoct in their kitchens the drugs that are going through the arduous approval process.

More recently, the Goldwater Institute has been spearheading the "Right to Try" legislation, which allows terminally ill patients to bypass the FDA and to negotiate directly with the drug companies to obtain medications not yet approved. Right to Try is passing state-by-state approval with an average support level of 90%. As of this writing, 38 states have implemented it (Goldwater Institute 2017). The US Congress is now considering it; as of this writing, the legislation has passed the Senate (US Congress 2017a).

Dr. Ebrahim Delpassand has treated 78 cancer patients under the Right to Try laws passed in Texas. Delpassand spent 5 years treating 150 patients with a drug that has been available in Europe for 15 years. In 2015, after the US study was successfully completed, the FDA refused to allow him to continue the treatments until the drug received the agency's approval. Right to Try allowed the desperate patients continued access to the drug (Goldwater Institute 2016).

Unfortunately, Right to Try has given only a relatively few patients relief. Drug companies are hesitant to work with patients directly for fear that the FDA will punish them for cutting the agency out of the loop. As long as FDA approvals are necessary for drug marketing, the agency holds the pharmaceutical firms—and patients—hostage.

Even the Defense Department, another government agency, recognizes that the FDA's approval authority is deadly. Section 732 of HR 2810—the National Defense Authorization Act for Fiscal Year 2018—originally proposed that the Secretary of Defense should be able to override the FDA's approval authority and use unapproved medical drugs and products for our troops overseas (US Congress 2017b). The FDA's 10-year refusal to approve freeze-dried plasma for emergency use by our soldiers has evidently created the frustration behind Section 732 (Diamond 2017).

While our troops are risking their lives to ensure our liberties, their medical freedom is being compromised by regulatory bureaucrats who are not legally liable for denying our military a potentially lifesaving medical product. Of course, the same bureaucrats are denying those of us at home freedom of choice as well. We will never have our medical freedom as long as regulators who do not have to experience the consequences of their choices get to decide our fate.

In spite of the wealth of evidence that the Amendments and the FDA approval process is a detriment to our health, some people will feel uncomfortable without an FDA sign off for the drugs they take. The FDA's drug and biologics division can be left in place to certify drugs (Chapter 50). Those who prefer the regulatory agency's input before they take a drug can have it. Those who prefer earlier access will have that too. That's the freedom our country was founded upon.

PASS THE HEALTH FREEDOM ACT HR 2117

In 2007, then-Representative Ron Paul of Texas introduced HR 2117, The Health Freedom Protection Act (US Congress 2017c), which basically countered the 2004 court decision that making a health claim for a food or nutrient turned it into a drug. Although this legislation did not pass, something similar to this bill might be necessary to keep the FDA from once again attempting to control information about natural products.

With repeal of the Amendments and the ability of the American public to purchase drugs at any stage of development, the FDA will have a much more difficult time limiting the public's access to foods and drugs that have utility in health and disease and any related information.

However, with the repeal of the Amendments, advertising for drugs and nutrients might revert to the Federal Trade Commission, where it once resided. Without passage of HR 2117 or something similar, another agency, possibly with the cooperation of the FDA, could begin to prosecute manufacturers that made dubious claims about their products.

Without the FDA policing ads, how would consumers know that they were getting accurate information? Certifying agencies, described in the next chapter, would likely take over that role. Instead of TV ads with exhaustive lists of side effects that cause listeners to zone out, ads would likely be more relevant. No certifying agency would want its name associated with false advertising, or it would quickly be out of business. Firms that made totally bogus claims for their products could still be prosecuted for false advertising, but the burden of proof would be on the accuser to show that the ad was truly fraudulent.

Without bureaucratic control of their health choices, patients would, we hope, make their choices in collaboration with trusted health care providers. If patients make a poor choice, they may die; if they make a good one, they may live or live better. Even the best drugs don't always work in everyone and can cause potentially deadly allergic reactions in some, so death is always an unfortunate possibility in any treatment selection. In the next chapter, we'll explore how to limit the risk of deadly side effects without the FDA approval process.

Chapter 50

Certification Is the Alternative to Regulation

I f the FDA didn't have the power to force new drugs and supplements through its long development process, we would expect more innovation. With more new drugs available, some of which are likely to be natural products, how will the average person and health care provider be able to discern which drugs are likely to help and which are likely to cause harm?

Certification is the tried and true way for protecting the consumer. Certification differs from regulation in that consumers, rather than regulators, make the ultimate decision on whether or not to buy and use a product.

Chapter 47 explained how excess regulation—such as licensing of optometrists, dentists, and electricians—lowers the amount of quality service delivered. By making service providers jump through costly and time-consuming regulatory hoops, the number of service providers is limited, and the service becomes so expensive that many consumers do without, thereby losing their health or even their lives. The reader will recognize that this process is happening with our pharmaceuticals today.

Certification, conversely, increases the number of service providers compared to places with stringent regulations or no regulations at all. More service providers can mean increased competition, which lowers prices and keeps products affordable. Overall, more quality service is delivered with certification (Carroll & Gaston 1981, 1983).

How does certification work? Professional or consumer groups give their "Seal of Approval," or favorable reviews, to products or service providers that meet their high standards. Conservative consumers use only goods and services that are recommended by certifiers. However, if for some reason, consumers want to use a product or service that carries no certification, they would be able to legally do so.

Although most people are unaware of it, our appliances and electrical hardware are not licensed or regulated by a government agency as drugs are. Instead, a private certifying company, Underwriters Laboratories Inc. (UL), does most of the actual testing of more than six billion products, and it grants its UL Seal of Approval to those that meet its exacting standards (Campbell 1997, 8–13). Manufacturers pay an evaluation fee to fund the testing. Rather than being adversarial, UL educates manufacturers about how they can make their products safer. The ultimate winner is the consumer.

This entire process is voluntary in most countries, including the United States. However, most retailers won't sell an appliance or electrical component without the UL assurance of quality. As a consequence, manufacturers routinely apply for UL certification.

What keeps UL honest and discourages it from simply selling its seal to any manufacturer who pays the price? Although UL is the most-trusted name in electronics certification, UL has competition. If UL starts certifying shoddy products and if consumers quit valuing UL's seal, manufacturers will stop getting their certification from UL. Instead, they will turn to certifications that consumers equate with high quality. Competition is a fierce regulator and is driven by consumer satisfaction. In today's society, with near instantaneous distribution of critical consumer reviews through the Internet, a good reputation or brand name is crucial.

If FDA approval becomes optional, third-party drug testing and certification is likely to become a more prominent feature in our consumer landscape. Indeed, having data produced by a third party, rather than the manufacturer, is likely to be more objective and less likely to overlook potential safety issues because of politics. Like the UL model, manufacturers and certifiers are more likely to work with each other, rather than against each other, to produce the best drug products possible.

Indeed, Europe uses such certifying bodies in its approval process. Medical device manufacturers pay a private device certifying body (DCB) to oversee their studies and recommend the products to the regulators for rapid approval. As a result, in the early 1990s, medical device approval in Europe took an average of 250 days compared with 820 days in the United States (Wilkerson Group 1996).

If DCBs can safely certify medical devices in Europe, surely similar organizations could evaluate pharmaceuticals. Like UL, which has certified electrical products longer than the FDA has been in existence, DCBs would profit only as long as consumers regarded their seal of approval highly. Thus, certifiers would have great incentive to ensure that dangerous or ineffective drugs did not come to market under their seal.

Indeed, some FDA scientists would likely decide that they could do a better job than the agency could do in giving patients and health care professionals guidance as to what the benefits and risks of new drugs are. Such entrepreneurial individuals might form some of the earliest companies to offer certification and expert guidance to those seeking reliable information about pharmaceuticals.

Drug certifiers wouldn't be starting from scratch, however. Certification was popular in the days before the FDA became the powerful agency it is today.

The Elixir Sulfanilamide incident demonstrated the importance of certification. Elixir Sulfanilamide contained a safe drug that was dissolved in a solvent that proved to be deadly. The new mixture was not tested before its sale in 1937. As a result, 107 people died, and the chemist who made the mixture committed suicide (Mihm 2007).

One of the most-prominent certifiers of that time was the American Medical Association (AMA), which provided both third-party testing and evaluation. Instead of relying on the studies performed by the drug companies, as the FDA does today, the AMA actually conducted its own experiments. Third-party testing such as the AMA provided was considered more objective than that done by the firm selling its product.

At the time of the Elixir Sulfanilamide disaster, the AMA had not yet evaluated the drug or given it the organization's seal of approval. Indeed, the AMA was asked to help discover what had caused the drug to be toxic and thus identified the solvent, diethylene glycol, as the culprit. Physicians who treated their patients only with drugs that had the AMA's seal avoided this tragedy (Nicholas 1937, 1531–39).

Before the Amendments, private organizations often provided their own evaluation to help consumers and their physicians learn about new drugs. Like the AMA, some groups, such as Consumers' Research, conducted their own testing. Physicians and pharmacists reported their evaluations in trade journals and lay publications (Jackson 1970, 20; Dowling 1970, 123–24; Burrow 1970, 113–15; Sonnedecker 1970, 105–06).

Books (Jackson 1970, 17–22) and magazines such as *Ladies' Home Journal* and *Collier's* (Wilson 1942, 22–23) alerted readers to the dangers of specific products. As early as 1904, the General Federation of Women's Clubs sent out thousands of letters, promoted lectures, and distributed information to educate the public about drug side effects (Wilson 1942, 27). As the standard of quality became FDA approval, those third-party reviews were marginalized. This trend was unfortunate, because third-party reviews are likely to be less politicized and more objective than either FDA or drug company evaluations would be.

Since 1959, the American Hospital Formulary Service (AHFS n.d.) has been reviewing both approved and off-label uses for drugs in its annual AHFS Drug Information volume and its interactive Drug Information Clinical Database. *The Medical Letter on Drugs and Therapeutics* provides peer-reviewed drug evaluations and is published by a nonprofit organization founded in 1958. This publication is supported by subscriptions and has no advertising, grants, or donations, thereby ensuring that its conflicts of interest, especially with the pharmaceutical industry, are minimized (Medical Letter n.d.).

If FDA approval were no longer needed for drug approval, health care providers would likely turn to such organizations and publications for the latest on new drugs and for off-label uses for old ones. When the gold standard for drugs is no longer FDA approval, those organizations are likely to proliferate and specialize as consumers and health care providers demand unbiased and less-politicized information on which to base their decisions.

Today, when a drug is first marketed, only the drug companies and the physicians who run their clinical studies have any hands-on experience with them. Should FDA approval become optional for new drug marketing, then third-party testing and drug certification that is similar to what we see with electrical appliances would likely emerge.

As a transition step, the FDA itself could become a certifying agency, instead of a regulatory one. The FDA would give its seal of approval to drugs it deems safe and effective, but patients—with the guidance of their trusted health care providers—would decide whether to take a drug that didn't have the agency's certification. Conservative patients and physicians might use only drugs that had the FDA seal; desperately ill patients and their physicians might use drugs without it. Instead of a one-size-fits-all regulatory approval, certification would allow those needing medical treatment to choose the amount of risk that they felt was warranted by their condition. Each person's choice would be honored. This is the freedom that our country was founded upon.

The solution, both for safety and for lower-cost, more available drugs, is to strip the FDA of its monopoly power over drugs and let any patient use any drug that a doctor is willing to prescribe. The FDA would then be a certifier of drugs, but not a regulator. Any drug not certified by the FDA would have to carry a warning label, similar to that on a cigarette package, saying: "WARNING: This drug has not been certified by the FDA."
—David R. Henderson, Hoover Institution, Stanford University

Indeed, consumer groups, such as the Abigail Alliance, are able to reliably predict which drugs will be effective years before they are approved by the FDA (Chapter 10). Although the Alliance doesn't give out a seal of approval, its evaluations are an important resource for cancer patients even today.

On the safety side, Public Citizens' newsletter titled *Worst Pills, Best Pills* has warned readers about 11 out of 20 dangerous, FDA-approved drugs an average of 3.3 years before they were withdrawn (Public Citizen's Health Research Group 2011). Clearly, consumer groups have a good track record of predicting which drugs work and which ones have safety problems years before their approval or withdrawal, respectively. Because the FDA is accountable to Congress and depends on the pharmaceutical industry's user fees, it must play politics to survive. The nation's health is too often a secondary consideration; both approvals and withdrawals are delayed, thus costing millions of lives.

Certification has already become a prominent feature in the less-regulated nutritional supplement industry, because some brands don't always contain the amount of active ingredient(s) indicated by the label. Although the FDA has the authority to take such products off the market, the agency does not usually do so. Consequently, certifying organizations, such as Good Housekeeping, Consumer Reports, and ConsumerLab.com, perform independent third-party testing on nutritional products to help guide buyers (ConsumerLab.com. n.d.). Consumers want to know that they are getting what they are paying for, so the certifiers provide the information by charging consumers a modest fee or by billing manufacturers for the testing, as UL does. Some consumers prefer certifiers who aren't paid by manufacturers and are willing to pay for this extra level of protection against possible corruption.

The Life Extension Foundation (LEF) has long used independent laboratory evaluation (third-party testing) for its house brand. In most cases, no seal of approval is given, but the ability of LEF to provide a testing report from a third party gives consumers confidence that what is on label is what is in the bottle. Third-party testing can thus provide an informal sort of certification.

LEF reviews the vast scientific literature to educate its customers about both benefits and potential side effects of nutritional supplements (LifeExtension n.d.). After the FDA's failure to imprison the founders of LEF, the agency has largely left that organization alone, which has allowed LEF to give its members leading edge nutritional and drug information (LEF 2017). Although I gather information from many sources, I have found LEF to be one of the few resources that I recommend to people looking for the latest on nutrients and cutting-edge therapies. Word-of-mouth recommendations, in addition to formal certifications, product reviews, and Internet commentary, are one more resource that both consumers and health care professionals can turn to when a government agency is not censoring information sharing.

Chapter 51

Drug Companies Rarely Profit by Selling Unsafe or Ineffective Drugs

Many critics of the drug industry believe that companies can profit by putting a dangerous product on the market, but that's rarely, if ever, the case. For example, Vioxx sales were, at most, around $10 Billion if we make the unrealistic assumption that maximum annual sales were made each year that it was on the market.[24] Merck's costs exceeded this amount: $6.6 billion in liability settlements (GoldenbergLaw PLLC n.d.; Wasseman 2016), $1.9 billion in paybacks to government entities for illegal marketing practices (Drug Watch 2016), $1 billion or more in development costs, close to $1 Billion in legal fees (Weiss 2008, 199), and $0.8 billion to investors enraged by the drop in Merck's stock price (Loftus 2016). Those losses alone totaled about $11.3 billion.[25]

The items just listed do not include the cost of the highly paid management time needed to deal with this disaster for more than a decade, the lost investment in the Vioxx production line, the inventory that could no longer be sold, and the plunging stock prices that exceeded reimbursements to investors.

In most pharmaceutical firms, stock options are a significant part of the compensation for high-level management. A Vioxx-like drug disaster would financially penalize the very people who decided to market it. Pharmaceutical firms and their employees have large incentives to make

sure that they don't put dangerous drugs on the market. However, being human, they will make mistakes, just as regulators—and the rest of
us—do.

Indeed, Vioxx was the most-dangerous drug ever put on the American market and was approved by the FDA under the Amendments (Chapter 31). Even though thalidomide was kept off US pharmacy shelves in
the 1960s by pre-Amendment regulations, the Amendments created an
American thalidomide incident by censoring information about how to
prevent neural tube defects with the B vitamin, folic acid (Chapter 34).

Today, FDA approval, not the manufacturer's track record, is the gold
standard. In a marketplace that didn't require FDA approval, the brand
name would be much more important as it was before passage of the
Amendments (Chapter 2). The loss in consumer confidence and, more
importantly, the confidence of prescribing physicians would be much
larger as well. Poisoning patients, along with the disastrous public image
that results, is bad for business. A company that did so with impunity
would be unlikely to survive long.

Many people fear that without FDA oversight, regardless of how expensive, cumbersome, and life-threatening it may be, a multitude of ineffective or dangerous drugs would come to market even though that has
not been the case historically. As earlier chapters have documented, the
marketplace generally protects the consumer from waste more effectively
than regulations do (Chapter 31). The savings created by the Amendments in keeping ineffective drugs off the market is more than offset by
the ever-increasing development costs and drug prices used to determine
efficacy.

Indeed, most of the studies show that pre-Amendment waste was
limited. Today, we have the Internet; virtually every product gets reviewed quickly by online consumers. Ineffective drugs, or those with un-
acceptable side effects, can be uncovered more quickly than ever before.

In spite of the strong evidence presented in this book and its demonstration that the 1962 Amendments are, quite literally, regulatory overkill, some people will still fear that allowing patients to buy drugs without

FDA approval will put us at the mercy of snake oil salesmen. Ironically, the much-maligned snake oil marketers may have been offering a worthwhile product. Snake oil is a revered dietary ingredient in oriental medicine. Like fatty fish, such as salmon, sea snake oil has high concentrations of omega-3 fatty acids, the building blocks of the good eicosanoids found in both prescription and over-the-counter fish oil. Rattlesnake oil, which was probably what most US snake oil actually was, has about half as much omega-3 as sea snake (Graber 2007), which is still a considerable amount. For folks who didn't take daily doses of cod liver oil, snake oil probably did contribute to overall health.

Snake oil, unlike fish oil, may also increase muscle endurance, something that would have been a great benefit in the early 20th century when most Americans were involved in heavy labor. Mice fed 6% sea snake oil were able to swim much longer than were mice on a 6% fish oil diet (Zhang, Shirai, Higuchi, et al. 2007, 476–81), suggesting that snake oil has something as yet unidentified that might be a beneficial dietary component.

Most folk medicine and herbal remedies that have withstood the test of time usually have healing properties. Indeed, most of our early drugs were based on such products, and many still are. Willow bark, made into a tea, was used by Native Americans as a pain reliever. The active ingredient, salicin, is converted to salicylic acid (a form of aspirin) in the body.

Chapter 52

Would Drug Development Change without FDA Approval?

I f FDA approval were not required to sell new drugs, how would the marketplace look? For the pharmaceutical giants, very little would change, at least at first. Those companies have learned to work with the regulators and to get approvals, even though the process is costly and time-consuming. Initially at least, the large drug firms would likely work with the FDA as they do now to obtain the agency's recommendation or certification, even though a drug could be marketed without those things.

Smaller companies, with perhaps a handful of drugs in their pipeline, would likely react differently. Because they are the actual source of many breakthrough drugs today, those firms would likely jump at the chance to sell their products to willing patients and to avoid the long years and costs of regulatory demands. The smaller companies would no longer have to hand off their discoveries to a pharmaceutical giant for the heavy lifting of Amendment-driven development. In addition, their products could get to market sooner, helping both patients and the smaller firm's bottom line.

An example of such a small biotech might be Sarepta, which is developing drugs for Duchenne's disease. Duchenne patients can't make the dystrophin protein, which is necessary for muscle growth. Children who can't make this protein eventually lose their ability to move—and breathe. One out of 3,600 male infants is born with this disease (MedlinePlus n.d.). At any one time, a couple of thousand boys in the United States need treatment to slow or stop the progression of the disease (Olsen 2015, 59).

Sarepta has 11 drugs in its development pipeline (Sarepta 2018), each targeting one of the several different genetic defects that cause Duchenne's. Sarepta's drugs cause the body to skip over those defects and produce shorter versions of the dystrophin protein. Eteplirsen, the drug that has been most-extensively tested, targets the defect at the "exon 51" site of mRNA, the genetic material that directs the body to make dystrophin. About 13% of Duchenne's patients are believed to have an exon 51 defect.

A British study was completed in June 2010 (Smart Patients n.d.), which demonstrated that eteplirsen did indeed increase levels of dystrophin in 7 out of 19 patients after 12 weeks of treatment (Cirak, Arechavala-Gomeza, Guglieri, et al. 2011, 595–605). In a second study that was done in the United States, 12 patients were treated with eteplirsen, and 4 received a placebo.

Halfway through the US study, Jenn McNary, who had two boys with Duchenne's, sought out Chris Garabedian, CEO of Sarepta. Even though the study was still blinded, Jenn confidently assured Chris that the drug worked. Her son, Max, who was in the trial, had gone from using a wheelchair half of the time to playing outside. He was able to open containers once again. His improvement on the drug was unheard of in Duchenne's patients (Olsen 2015, 40). After 48 weeks on eteplirsen, Duchenne boys were walking 21 meters farther than they had at the start of the study and 68 meters farther than those receiving placebo. The placebo patients were immediately switched to eteplirsen, because it was considered unethical to deprive them of this potentially lifesaving treatment (Sarepta Therapeutics 2012).

Jenn's other son, Austin, had been excluded from the trial. Jenn pleaded with Chris to let Austin take the drug too, because he was continuing to deteriorate.

Chris explained the difficult situation: Sarepta had only enough of the drug to treat the patients in the clinical study. The only way investors would put up more money, which would allow Sarepta to manufacture more of the drug, was if the FDA showed interest in approving it.

The trial results were announced in early October 2012. By 2014, improvements in lung function, rather than the expected deterioration, were seen in the etiplirsen-treated boys after more than 2 years of treatment (Sarepta Therapeutics 2014).

Because the drug wasn't showing any troubling side effects in the boys, eteplirsen could likely have been marketed before the Amendments. After all, it had been demonstrated to be safe for the intended use. Under the Amendments, however, the FDA continued to insist on more rigorous effectiveness testing, even though Duchenne's is essentially an orphan disease and could enjoy accelerated approval based on smaller clinical trials. Instead, the FDA demanded more muscle biopsies of the treated children to get better statistical data showing that dystrophin is indeed increased. The biopsy required anesthetizing the boys and cutting out a piece of muscle, the very tissue that is slow to regrow.

Our children can no longer be your science experiment. The children are not here to serve science. The science should always serve the children.
—Mariss Penrod, mother of a Duchenne child, addressing the FDA

Meanwhile, thousands of boys face this crippling disease knowing that a drug that might help them is being withheld from them. Austin McNary, brother to Max, was one of those children (Olsen 2015, 37). While Max got better, Austin got worse. Jenn helped to organize the Duchenne community to pressure the FDA to approve eteplirsen, but the FDA kept refusing to do so.

Finally, the FDA suggested a safety trial on the older, sicker Duchenne boys, including Austin. His mother, Jenn, thinks that the FDA was trying to placate the Duchenne community so they would stop badgering it. That didn't happen.

Chris Garabedian, who was unpopular with the FDA, resigned from the Sarapeta board and his position as CEO in March 2015 in an attempt to pacify the agency (Chen & Burger 2015). In April 2016, however, the FDA once again refused to approve eteplirsen.

In September 2016, a British study with another Sarepta Duchenne drug—this one targeting the exon-53 defect—showed statically signif-icant increases in dystrophen for all of the boys treated for 48 weeks (Sarepta Therapeutics 2017). A couple of weeks later, the FDA finally re-lented and gave accelerated approval to eteplirsen, now called Exondys 51, on the condition that Sarepta perform additional studies demonstrat-ing improvement in motor function in those receiving the drug. If the agency is unsatisfied with results, it may withdraw the Exondys 51 from the market (US FDA 2016).

If the FDA approval was not needed for the sale of drugs, eteplirsen would likely have been on the market years earlier, and the drug target-ing the Exon-53 defect might be available today as well. Investors would have gladly put up the money to manufacture and sell eteplirsen, and the Duchenne community would have been thrilled to purchase it. Who wouldn't want to try a drug that was reversing the crippling of Duchenne's disease in at least some children? Best of all, the drug would likely cost about a fraction of its current cost if it could have been marketed in 2012.

With eteplirsen on the market, Sarepta and other companies would have incentive to develop drugs that would help some of the other 87% of the Duchenne's sufferers. Those lifesaving drugs have already been identified, but the FDA's foot-dragging has discouraged investors from putting up the money for their development.

Even if FDA approval were not required for marketing, some insurers might elect not to pay for drugs that did not have FDA certification or recommendation. Because the development time for new, unapproved drugs would be less costly in time and money, prices would be pro-portionately lower. Many patients could probably afford them, even if their insurance didn't cover them. However, if the drugs performed well, insurers would find it less costly to pay for them than for the medical alternatives. A wheelchair-bound Duchene's child would be much more expensive to insurers, for example, than is one who is able to continue walking.

Insurers who wouldn't pay for an effective treatment might be successfully sued by their policyholders. Courts have already ruled in favor of some of Burzynski's patients when "incurable" brain cancers went into remission, even if insurance companies balked because his treatment wasn't "usual and customary" (i.e., FDA approved) (Ausubel 2000, 261).

Once insurers start paying for new drugs that are not certified by the FDA, even the large pharmaceutical firms are likely to abandon the regulatory route unless the FDA takes drastic measures to streamline the red tape. The competition from an alternative path to the marketplace will create incentives for the FDA to meet consumer demands for earlier access to new drugs. The best way to reform the agency is to make it compete for the respect of the medical, pharmaceutical, and patient community. Ironically, the FDA regulators are likely to take less heat from legislators when the inevitable side effects do arise, because drugs can come to the market without the Amendment-driven provision that they sign off on approvals.

Without the Amendments, many of the legislative bandages that were put in place to alleviate problems caused by the Amendments would no longer be necessary. PDUFA-driven user fees would be lower or nonexistent, because FDA certification wouldn't be necessary for marketing. The 7-year monopoly that drug companies received for Orphan Drug status would no longer be available, because there would be no more approvals. Moreover, development costs would be lower without the Amendments, and fewer drugs would be orphans; many more would be able to recover the less-intensive development costs. The Waxman Hatch Patent Restoration Act wouldn't add to the patent life of drugs because clinical development times would plummet.

Instead of doing large human trials to get statically significant results, drug companies would focus on smaller trials designed to determine which patients respond best to their potential new product. This approach will allow companies to target their product toward those who will actually benefit. Because patients will be taking fewer drugs that "might" help them, the incidence of drug–drug interactions will decrease. Deaths from "properly prescribed medications," which now rank close to the fifth largest cause of death, should decrease too. Although the technology to determine who will benefit most from a particular drug is often available, pharmaceutical firms must focus instead on the outdated studies demanded by the FDA (Huber 2013).

People who fear that earlier access might mean less safety could elect to take only drugs that have FDA certification, even though drugs could be marketed without it. Patients who want earlier access could also have it. People could choose for themselves. That is the freedom upon which our country was founded.

As the marketplace adjusted to the less-intensive regulatory climate, we would see more innovation, both in pharmaceuticals and nutraceuticals. Without the Amendments, the FDA could not pose restrictions on what manufacturers' representatives could say to doctors. Supplement suppliers could educate physicians on the benefits of using natural products (e.g., vitamins) instead of drugs. Pharmaceutical firms would be able to combine their drugs with CoQ10 and other nutrients to lessen side effects. Instead of being at odds, drug companies and nutraceutical firms might find it profitable to collaborate on research, marketing, or product design.

Without the FDA's ability to damper prevention through the use of natural products or to combine them with pharmaceuticals to lessen side effects, physicians would likely become more knowledgeable about prevention. This approach will help the American public become healthier as well.

Because about two-thirds of the American populace is currently overweight, drug companies need not worry that they will run out of people who need treatment. Unfortunately, many people won't take the initiative to eat less, exercise more, or do other things to promote their own well-being, even after being diagnosed with diabetes, cardiovascular disease, and other lifestyle dependent maladies. Many will continue to prefer drugs to lifestyle changes or will find that we don't know enough about prevention to control their disease without drugs.

Without the FDA able to treat stem cell products as drugs that need to go through an intensive development program before those in need can benefit, stem cell research will return to the United States, making it much more affordable. Individual physicians will no longer have to worry about continuously being hauled into court simply because they have not checked all the regulatory boxes required by a bureaucratic development plan. Parents will not have to beg the agency to allow their children to try new treatments that might save their lives or keep them out of wheelchairs.

In short, we will once again be poised on a Golden Age of Health as we were in the early 1960s. However, this time we will have better science, more know-how, and a better understanding of what spurs innovation and what squelches it.

However, the proposed changes will be difficult to implement. Many regulators will not want to give up their approval power, even though lifesaving drugs will be more available for themselves and their loved ones when consumers are free to choose. Pharmaceutical firms won't dare support less regulation as long as the FDA has the power to destroy them at will. Legislators will fear that they will be criticized by voters who equate long, drawn-out development plans with safety and effectiveness if they allow drugs not approved by the FDA to be marketed.

If we are to regain the freedom to save our lives with supplements, drugs, or other medical procedures of our choice, the effort must come from you, dear reader. If you want to live longer and better, you must take action.

Never doubt that a small group of committed, thoughtful citizens can change the world. Indeed, it's the only thing that ever has.
—Margaret Mead, American anthropologist

What should this action be? Put your individual talent and knowledge toward restoring our medical freedom. We all have contributions to make. Perhaps we can at long last reclaim our Golden Age of Health that was thwarted by the 1962 Amendments.

Afterword

S o now we know! Dr. Mary Ruwart has done us all a big favor. Not only has she has identified a huge problem that is affecting the well-being of millions of people, but also she's laid out the history, proof, and many touching and illustrative human stories that demonstrate a truly viable solution to part of our health crisis. Even more important, she has charted a course to reverse the damage, and she has identified the principles and the path by which millions more can be empowered in their health.

In the THRIVE Movie and Movement, we make our best efforts to assist people with critical thinking about how to understand and solve the key issues that are threatening us. Again and again, the pattern comes back to revealing that our major problems are breakdowns in the wholeness of natural systems. So we need to learn what a healthy living system looks like and to discover the compass by which we can restore wholeness. This is just what Ruwart has done.

Death by Regulation is a useful and admirable model for exactly how to do this from an expert in both honest science and true freedom. If we are simply grateful and impressed by what Ruwart has done, we will have missed the real point of her writing this book. Her offering is a shining example of excellent investigative reporting, and—just as much—it's a graceful kick in the butt to each of us to wake up and take action, whether on this particular issue or on countless related others.

The author has demonstrated that centralized control leads to a monopoly of power and to inevitable corruption. She gets to the heart of the matter for solving the deadly delays and bias in the pharmaceutical industry by returning to first principles—to the innate right of all individuals to choose their actions as long as they are not coercing or harming anyone else. By extension, this action leads to a true free market of voluntary exchange with individual accountability for everyone.

Ruwart has clearly shown how the 1962 "Amendments" put small pharmaceutical firms out of business; stifled about 80% of innovations; led to shorter lives, higher health care costs, and more corruption; and shifted the paradigm from prevention to treatment. Even more tragically, she cites that 15 million people had died by 2009 due solely to the delays caused by those onerous regulations in getting drugs from the lab bench to the market. More have died than the number of Americans killed in all US wars!

So is this mass destruction due to mere incompetence? Ruwart sticks to her areas of expertise in science, pharmaceuticals, and liberty. After decades of connecting the dots across sectors and around the world, however, I personally recommend that we consider larger and deeper motivations, so that we know better what we are up against as we are looking to rectify this problem and create viable solutions that are truly commensurate with the challenges we face. This book has pointed out the motivation of greed and the strategy of control. I would add this question: *toward what end?* Of course, there's a huge financial incentive to maximize profit, but if we truly follow the money, as we did in THRIVE, we will discover that the same individuals, families, and controlling financial institutions are behind similar takeovers in all sectors—including education, media, energy, food, and—of course—money itself. These are the very powers that have been systematically increasing our national debt and inflating our currency, so it behooves us to look beyond the payoff to the agenda of control, not only of the United States, but also of all regions in the globalist strategy for domination.

While this is my conclusion, rather than Ruwart's, we both agree on the solution: more freedom, not less. Those who wish to control us have become adept at convincing the public that less freedom means more safety, security, and comfort when, in fact, the opposite is true.

Dr. Benjamin Rush, one of the signers of the Declaration of Independence, reputedly warned: "Unless we put medical freedom into the Constitution, the time will come when medicine will organize into an undercover dictatorship. To restrict the art of healing to one class of men, & deny equal privileges to others, will be to constitute the Bastille of medical science. All such laws are un-American and despotic, & have no place in a Republic."

As Ruwart has demonstrated, the Amendments have helped to institute that medical dictatorship. Terminally ill Americans are forbidden to save their lives with drugs that haven't yet been approved by the bureaucratic FDA. Physicians with new ideas, such as Stanislaw Burzynski, are persecuted and prosecuted.

The antidote to such evil is to do away with the lethal belief in authoritarian rule of a few over others and to reclaim our natural right to govern ourselves. Ruwart's extensive background in moral philosophy, the Non-Aggression principle, and its practical application (see her *Healing Our World* and *Short Answers to the Tough Questions*) informs her profound analysis of what we can do and how it could and would work.

Ruwart shows how "certification" is the healthy alternative to oppressive regulation. She reminds us that patients should make their decisions because they are the ones that must experience the consequences.

So what are we to do? In the THRIVE Movement, we teach a "whole systems" solutions model where local or virtual communities can organize activist initiatives to coordinate expertise in all sectors. Such initiatives go around the principles of liberty and toward restoring the wholeness of voluntary exchange and individual accountability.

When Dr. Mary Ruwart was deeply impacted by the tragic truths she was learning about the state of pharmaceuticals in the United States, she set out to do something about it. This remarkable book is her offering. What we take from it to apply to this and other important issues is our gift back to her and forward to our fellow humans. Onward!

Foster Gamble
Co-creator, THRIVE Movie and Movement
http://www.thrivemovement.com/

Acknowledgments

T his book would not be possible without the work of hundreds of researchers, each of whom has allowed me to document the horrifying impact of the 1962 Amendments. My role has been to take their contributions and point out the implications, thereby painting the picture of the immense death and suffering created by those regulations.

Although early investigators, such as Sam Peltzman and Dale Gieringer had shown that the benefits of the Amendments were far outweighed by their costs, I did not anticipate just how deadly they really were. Because what happens in the United States ripples outward, the entire world has been adversely affected by this legislation. I owe special thanks to those two investigators and to Jerome Schnee, whose work on pre-Amendment development times provided crucial insight into the deadly delays created by the regulations. Had I been unaware of the contributions of those three researchers, I might never have written *Death by Regulation*.

In addition, I would like to particularly acknowledge the work of Ronald Hansen, Henry Grabowski, and Joseph DiMasi. Without their dedicated work over the past several decades, we might be unaware of just how much the cost of bringing a new drug to market has risen and continues to rise.

I want to give special thanks to Frank Lichtenberg for sharing with me his compilation of approved and withdrawn drugs, as well as his work in estimating how many lives the average new drug saves. Because *Death by Regulation* focuses on the impact of the 1962 Amendments, only a small portion of Lichtenberg's vast research on the impact of pharmaceuticals was cited herein.

Moreover, I have made every effort to represent the research of those and the many other cited individuals as appropriately as possible. Any mistakes or misrepresentations are mine alone.

I am immensely grateful to Ron Paul, Jonathan Wright, and Foster Gamble for their foreword, preface, and afterword respectively. As a congressman, Ron Paul saw how regulations thwarted the supplement industry; Jonathan Wright experienced the heavy hand of the Food and Drug Administration (FDA) directly when it raided his clinic. Foster Gamble "follows the money" and takes his investigations a step further than I do here. Each comes from a perspective that helps the reader appreciate the further implications of *Death by Regulation*.

Several of my Upjohn colleagues, notably Duane Lakings, Bob Rush, and Karen Wilkinson, have given me invaluable advice and suggestions for this manuscript. Several other reviewers who made significant contributions were Justin Arman, James Lark, Bartley Madden, Howard Meyers, Teresa Post, Ken Schoolland, and Karen Swindell. Their collective input improved the book immeasurably.

I was delighted to work again with my editor, Barbara Hart, and her talented team from Publications Professionals. Judy O'Brien and her group at Hasmark provided the cover art and sorely needed pre-market preparation and advice. This book would not be possible without the help of such professionals.

Potential Conflicts of Interest: Although this book was not funded directly by the pharmaceutical industry, I was supported by savings and retirement funds from my time at the Upjohn Company, as well as my work as chair of a for-profit IRB (Institutional Review Board). I have, in the past, been a consultant and writer for the Life Extension

Foundation and an expert witness against the FDA. In *Death by Regulation*, I describe the FDA's raids and legal action against Jonathan Wright and Bill Faloon, both of whom I know personally. I am also a supporter of Barry Sears and his landmark research on the anti-inflammatory effects of fish oil and the Zone Diet, as well as the Goldwater Institute's Right to Try legislation.

Endnotes

1. Pre-Amendment development times for self-originated and acquired new drugs were taken from Schnee (1970). Development times were adjusted by the author to reflect a mixture of 78% self-originated new drugs and 22% acquired new drugs to correspond to the post-Amendment data.

2. The 1963–99 post-Amendment development times were taken directly from DiMasi (2001a), which reported a mixture of 78% self-originated new drugs and 22% acquired new drugs. The estimate of the 2000–09 development times was made as follows: The 1990s development time for self-originated new drugs was 11.8 years as per DiMasi, Hansen, and Grabowski (2003). The 2000s development time for self-originated drugs was 10.7 years as per DiMasi, Grabowski, and Hansen (2016). The difference between the two time periods was 1.1 years (11.8 years – 10.7 years). If we assume that acquired new drugs in the 2000s enjoyed the same decrease in development time from the 1990s as self-originated ones, the estimated development times for the 2000s would be 13.1 years (14.2 years – 1.1 years).

3. The figure shows a mixture of 78% self-originated drugs (those discovered by the developing company) and 22% acquired ones (those discovered by an entity other than the developer). Acquired drugs generally take longer to get to market because the time to negotiate a licensing agreement can greatly extend development time. The transition year 1962 is not included.

4. The weighted average for years of life lost to heart disease (11 years) and to stroke (10 years) is 10.8 years. Using 11 years instead of 10.8 years gives a slightly more conservative estimate of lives lost.

5. List compiled from Freedom of Information requests by FR Lichtenberg and from the FDA website by author. See US FDA n.d.b.

6. JA DiMasi (2001a) as displayed in Figure 1.

7. Mean development time minus the pre-Amendment development time of 4 years as displayed in Figure 1.

8. Years caused by the Amendments multiplied by the 18,800 life-years each drug presumably saved in 1991, as per Lichtenberg (2003). An adjustment was also made for the population during the appropriate decade from the 1960s to the 2000s (0.78, 0.85, 0.94, 1.04, and 1.14, respectively).

9. Obtained by dividing life-years lost by 11 years, the average years of life lost to heart disease in 1991 as per Lichtenberg (2003) and US Census (2012a).

10. Page 374 estimates an age-adjusted drop in heart attack mortality of 40% from 1975 to 1995. Because 1975 deaths were 757,000, a 40% drop in 1995 would save 302,800 lives. Page 376 estimates that 27.5% of this decline is due to aspirin, which means that that drug saved about 83,230 lives per year. A delay of 20 years would result in 1.7 million lives lost.

11. Data taken from Hansen (1979); DiMasi, Hansen, Grabowski, et al. (1991); DiMasi, Hansen, Grabowski (2003); DiMasi & Grabowski (2007); and DiMasi, Grabowski, & Hansen (2016) and converted to 2015 $ by the author.

12. Calculated from data taken from Schnee (1970) and MN Baily (1972) and converted to 2015 $ by the author.

13. The pre-Amendment trend (broken lines) is an extrapolation from the decade prior to the Amendments until 2008.

14. Those figures were calculated using Microsoft Excel 2007.

15. The average price for a branded prescription drug was taken from Eli Lilly Company (1972, 24) and US Census Bureau (2012b, 113, Table 159) and converted to 2015 dollars by author.

16. Pre-Amendment capitalized R&D/NCE was calculated by author from data taken from Schnee (1970) and Baily (1972).

17. Post-Amendment R&D/NCE was taken from Hansen (1979); DiMasi, Hansen, Grabowski, et al. (1991); DiMasi, Hansen, Grabowski (2003); DiMasi & Grabowski (2007); and DiMasi, Grabowski, & Hansen (2016) and converted to 2015 $ by the author.

18. The extrapolations are by the author; the 10.1% capitalization rate is based on the average rate for 2005 and 2010 in Table 3 from DiMasi, Grabowski, & Hansen 2016.

19. The $50 estimate is from author's query from two compounding pharmacies in 2016.

20. Data are from Peltzman (1973). Reformatted and colorized by FDAReview.org, a project of the Independent Institute and reprinted with permission. http://www.fdareview.org/05_harm.php, acc. July 10, 2017.

21. From the weighted average of life years lost from heart disease and cerebrovasular disease in 1997 taken from US Census Bureau (2004, Table No. 112), which translates to about 109,090 lives saved per NCE (1,080,000 life-years divided by 11 life-years per life saved = 98,182 lives saved per NCE over its lifetime).

22. Gieringer 1985.

23. Estimated by sponsors of the Health Freedom Protection Act (HR 4282) in Faloon (2011, 218).

24. Merck & Co., Inc. Annual Report 2003, page 19, indicates $2.4 billion in sales, with a 2% increase over 2002 at http://www.merck.com/finance/annualreport/ar2003/pdf/mer-

ck2003ar.pdf, acc. February 3, 2017. If we assume that sales were at this level from its launch in May 1999 to its withdrawal in September 2004, maximum sales were about $10 billion. This estimate is likely high, because it takes several years for sales of a new drug to peak.

25. For 1997 approvals, the capitalized cost of new drug development was $802 million (2000 dollars), according to DiMasi, Hansen, & Grabowski, et al. (2003). Extrapolating to 1999 (see Figure 2), an approval would be close to $1 billion. Vioxx's development cost probably exceeded that, as it had some of the largest Phase 3 trials ever performed in the 20th century.

References

Abelson, R, & A Pollack. 2001. Other Drugs to Combat Anthrax Are in Ample Supply. *New York Times*, Oct. 23, B8.

Adams, M. 2007. Tyranny in the USA: The True History of FDA Raids on Healers, Vitamin Shops, and Supplement Companies. Apr. 12. https://www.naturalnews.com/021791.html, acc. Mar. 15, 2016.

Adams, PA, & VV Brantner. 2006. Estimating the Cost of New Drug Development: Is It Really $802 Million? *Health Affairs*, Mar.–Apr.;25(2): 420–28.

Aiken, JW, RR Gorman, & RJ Shebuski. 1979. Prevention of Blockage of Partially Obstructed Coronary Arteries with Prostacyclin Correlates with Inhibition of Platelet Aggregation. *Prostaglandins*, Apr;17(4): 483–94.

Algra, AM, & PM Rothwell. 2012. Effects of Regular Aspirin on Long-Term Cancer Incidence and Metastasis: A Systematic Comparison of Evidence from Observational Studies Versus Randomized Trials. *The Lancet Oncology*, 13(5): 518–27.

Allison, M. 2012. Reinventing Clinical Trials. *Nature Biotechnology*, Jan. 9;30(1): 41–49.

Altman, LK. 1987. Drug Seems to Halt an Infection Caused by the AIDS Virus. *New York Times*, Jan. 10. http://www.nytimes.com/1987/01/10/us/drug-seems-to-halt-an-infection-caused-by-the-aids-virus.html?pagewanted=all, acc. May 22, 2016.

American Hospital Formulary Service (AHFS). n.d. Homepage. http://www.ahfs-druginformation.com/, acc. Sep. 10, 2016.

American Society of Plastic Surgeons. 2016. New Statistics Reflect the Changing Face of Plastic Surgery. http://www.plasticsurgery.org/news/press-releases/new-statistics-reflect-the-changing-face-of-plastic-surgery, acc. Oct. 2, 2016.

Androgel®. 2007. Package insert. https://www.androgelpro.com/?cid=ppc_ppd_andro_ggl_brnd_5538, acc. Feb. 28, 2018.

Antiplatelet Trialists' Collaboration. 1994. Collaborative Overview of Randomized Trials of Antiplatelet Therapy–I: Prevention of Death, Myocardial Infarction, and Stroke by Prolonged Antiplatelet Therapy in Various Categories of Patients. *British Medical Journal*, Jan. 8;308(6921): 81–106.

AREDS2 (Age-Related Eye Diseases Study 2 Research Group). 2013. Lutein and Zeaxanthin and Omega 3 Fatty Acids for Age-Related Macular Degeneration, the Age-Related Eye Disease Study 2 (AREDS2) Randomized Clinical Trial. *Journal of the American Medical Association*, May 15;309(19): 2005–15.

Arhangelsky, P. 2011. Dietary Ingredients. July 1. http://emord.com/blawg/fda-publishes-draft-guidance-on-new-dietary-ingredients/, acc. Jan. 29, 2017.

Armstrong, GL, LA Conn, & RW Pinner. 1999. Trends in Infectious Disease Mortality in the United States during the 20th Century. *Journal of the American Medical Association*, Jan. 6;281(1): 61–66.

Arthur D Little Inc. 1984. Cost-Effectiveness of Pharmaceuticals #7: Beta-Blocker Reduction of Mortality and Reinfarction Rate in Survivors of Myocardial Infarction: A Cost-Benefit Study. (Washington, DC: Pharmaceutical Manufacturers Association), I.

Associated Press. 2001. Government Threatens to Suspend Patent on Cipro. *USA Today*, Oct. 23. http://usatoday30.usatoday.com/news/attack/2001/10/23/anthrax-cipro.htm, acc. May 21, 2016.

Atik, E, JA Gutierrez, FJL Filho, et al. 1989. Infusion of Prostaglandin E1 in Ductus-Dependent Congenital Heart Diseases. Analysis of 47 Cases. *Arquivos Brasileiros de Cardiologia*, Aug.;53(2): 93–97.

Austrian, R, & J Gold. 1964. Pneumococcal Bacteremia with Especial Reference to Bacteremic Pneumococcal Pneumonia. *Annals of Internal Medicine*, May;60(5): 759–76.

Ausubel, K. 2000. *When Healing Becomes a Crime: The Amazing Story of the Hoxsey Cancer Clinics and the Return of Alternative Therapies*. (Rochester, VT: Healing Arts Press), 118–34, 261.

BBC. 2014. Thalidomide: The Fifty-Year Fight. May 15. http://www.dailymotion.com/video/x3f1r17, acc. Mar. 30, 2017.

Baily, MN. 1972. Research and Development Costs and Returns: The US Pharmaceutical Industry. *Journal of Political Economy*, Jan.–Feb.;80(1): 70–85.

Bakke, OM, MA Manocchia, F de Abajo, et al. 1995. Drug Safety Discontinuations in the United Kingdom, the United States, and Spain from 1974 through

1993: A Regulatory Perspective. *Clinical Pharmacology and Therapeutics*, Aug.;58(1): 108–17.

Bakke, OM, WM Wardell, & L Lasagna. 1984. Drug Discontinuations in the United Kingdom and the United States, 1964–1983. *Issues of Safety, Clinical Pharmacology, and Therapeutics*, May;35(5): 559–67.

Baniasadi, S, P Eftekhari, P Tabarsi, et al. 2010. Protective Effect of N-Acetylcysteine on Anti-Tuberculosis Drug-Induced Hepatotoxicity. *European Journal of Gastroenterology and Hepatology*, Oct.;22(10): 1235–38.

Barber, M., AAC Dutton, MA Beard, et al. 1960. Reversal of Antibiotic Resistance in Hospital Staphylococcal Infection. *British Medical Journal*, Jan. 2;1(5165): 11–17.

Barcus, HA. 2010. When Does Medical Negligence Become Criminal? http://www .latlaw.com/index.php/firm-news-articles/articles-2010/88-when-does -medical-negligence-become-criminal, acc. July 4, 2016.

Barlas, S. 2014. Generic Prices Take Flight; The FDA Is Struggling to Ground Them. *Pharmacology and Therapeutics*, Dec.;39(12): 833, 843–45.

Barré-Sinoussi, F, JC Chermann, F Rey, et al. 1983. Isolation of a T-Lymphotropic Retrovirus from a Patient at Risk for Acquired Immune Deficiency Syndrome (AIDS). *Science*, May 20;220(4599): 868–71.

Beales, JH. 1996. New Uses for Old Drugs. In *Competitive Strategies in the Pharmaceutical Industry*, ed. RB Helms. (Washington, DC: American Enterprise Institute Press), 281–305. https://www.aei.org/wp-content/uploads/1996/06/Competitive -Strategies-In-The-Pharmaceutical-Industry-text.pdf, acc. Sep. 17, 2017.

Berger, JS, MC Roncaglioni, F Avanzini, et al. 2006. Aspirin for the Primary Prevention of Cardiovascular Events in Women and Men: A Sex-Specific Meta-Analysis of Randomized Controlled Trials. *Journal of the American Medical Society*, Jan. 18;295(3): 306–13.

Berkman, L. 1990. Ribavirin Fight Puts ICN on Ropes: Pharmaceuticals: Company Founder Milan Panic Said He Decided to Give Up the Battle with the FDA Because He Felt That There Was No Way He Could Win. *Los Angeles Times*, Mar. 2. http://articles.latimes.com/1990-03-02/business/fi-1816_1 _milan-panic, acc. May 21, 2016.

Berndt, ER, AHB Gottschalk, TJ Philipson, et al. 2005. Industry Funding of the FDA: Effects of PDUFA on Approval Times and Withdrawal Rates. *Nature Reviews/Drug Discovery*, July;4(7): 547–51.

Bhattacharya, S. 2005. Up to 140,000 Heart Attacks Linked to Vioxx. *New Scientist*, Jan. 25. https://www.newscientist.com/article/dn6918-up-to-140000-heart -attacks-linked-to-vioxx/, acc. Oct. 31, 2017.

Bojić, I, V Begović, P Mijuskovi, et al. 1995. Treatment of Patients with Subfulminant Forms of Viral Hepatitis B using Prostaglandin E1[translation;]. *Vojnosanitetski Pregled*, Sep–Oct.;52(5): 471–75.

Bond, RS, & DF Lean. 1977. Sales, Promotion, and Product Differentiation in Two Prescription Drug Markets. (Washington, DC: Bureau of Economics).

Borissova, AM, T Tankova, G Kirilov, et al. 2003. The Effect of Vitamin D3 on Insulin Secretion and Peripheral Insulin Sensitivity in Type 2 Diabetic Patients. *International Journal of Clinical Practice*, May;57(4): 258–56.

Boston Consulting Group. 1993. The Contribution of Pharmaceutical Companies: What's at Stake for America. (Boston: BCG).

Botting, J. 2015. *The History of Thalidomide, Animals, and Medicine: The Contribution of Animal Experiments to the Control of Disease.* (Cambridge, UK: Open Book Publishers), 183–98.

Bozzette, SA, G Joyce, DF McCaffrey, et al. 2001. HIV Cost and Services Utilization Study Consortium. Expenditures for the Care of HIV-Infected Patients in the Era of Highly Active Antiretroviral Therapy. *New England Journal of Medicine,* Mar. 15;344(11): 817–23.

Bren, L. 2001. Frances Oldham Kelsey: FDA Medical Reviewer Leaves Her Mark on History. https://web.archive.org/web/20090512235601/http://www.fda.gov/fdac/features/2001/201_kelsey.html, acc. Oct. 15, 2017.

Brickley, P, & R Winslow. 2014. Dendreon to Pursue Sale or Reorganization in Bankruptcy: Cancer-Treatment Maker Says Provenge Drug Will Remain Available. *Wall Street Journal,* Nov. 10. https://www.wsj.com/articles/dendreon-cancer-drug-maker-files-for-chapter-11-bankruptcy-1415609407, acc. Oct. 31, 2017.

Brimelow, P, & L Spencer. 1993. Food and Drugs and Politics. *Forbes Magazine,* Nov. 22, 116.

Burch, PA, JK Breen, JC Buckner, et al. 2000. Priming Tissue-Specific Cellular Immunity in a Phase 1 Trial of Autologous Dendritic Cells for Prostate Cancer. *Clinical Cancer Research,* Jun.;6(6): 2175–82.

Burdick, RE. 1997. Letter to Judge S Lake. Feb. 19. http://burzynskimovie.com/images/stories/transcript/Documents/1997BurdickLtr_Burzynski.pdf.

Burkholz, H. 1994. The FDA Follies: An Alarming Look at Our Food and Drugs in the 1980s. (New York: Basic Books): 113–22.

Burrow, JG. 1970. The Prescription Drug Policies of the American Medical Association in the Progressive Era. In *Safeguarding the Public: Historical Aspects of Medicinal Drug Control,* ed. JB Blake. (Baltimore: Johns Hopkins University Press), 113–15.

Burton, TM. 2002. Lilly Posts 20% Profit Decline, Warns of Product-Launch Delays. *Wall Street Journal*, July 19.

Burzynski, SR. 1976. Antineoplastons: Biochemical Defense Against Cancer. *Physiological Chemistry and Physics*, Mar.;8(3): 275–79.

———. 1977. Letter from Caldwell and Baggott, Attorneys at Law. June 21. http://www.burzynskimovie.com/images/stories/transcript/Documents /1977-06-21CaldwellandBaggott.pdf, acc. Oct. 31, 2017.

———. 1995. Burzynski: The Movie. http://www.burzynskimovie.com, acc. Mar. 6, 2016.

Calfee, JE. 1997. *Fear of Persuasion: A New Perspective on Advertising and Regulation*. (Monnaz, Switzerland: Agora Association with American Enterprise Institute for Public Policy Research).

Campbell, ND. 1997. Replace FDA Regulation of Medical Devices with Third-Party Certification. *Cato Policy Analysis*, No. 288, Nov. 12, 8–13.

Cantor, DJ. 1997. Prescription Drug User Fee Act of 1992: Effects on Bringing New Drugs to Market. CRS Report for Congress 97-838 E, Sep. 12. http://www.law .umaryland.edu/marshall/crsreports/crsdocuments/97-838_E.pdf, acc. Aug. 24, 2017.

Carlberg, C, S Seuter, VDF de Mello, et al. 2013. Primary Vitamin D Target Genes Allow a Categorization of Possible Benefits of Vitamin D3 Supplementation. PLOS ONE, Jul. 29;8(7): e71042.

Carroll, SL, & RJ Gaston. 1981. Occupational Restrictions and the Quality of Service Received: Some Evidence. *Southern Economic Journal*, Oct;47(4): 959–76.

———. 1983. Occupational Restrictions and the Quality of Service Received: An Overview. *Law and Human Behavior*, Sep.;7(2-3): 139–46.

Centeno, CJ. 2012. The Stem Cells They Don't Want You to Have: How the Stem Cell Debate Will Shape the Future of Medicine. p. 17. https://www.regenexx .com, acc. Oct. 12, 2017.

Centers for Disease Control (CDC). n.d. Leading Causes of Death, 1900–1998. http://www.cdc.gov/nchs/data/dvs/lead1900_98.pdf, acc. Apr. 6, 2014.

Chan, AT, N Arber, J Burn, et al. 2012. Aspirin in the Chemoprevention of Colorectal Neoplasia: An Overview. *Cancer Prevention Research (Philadelphia)*, Feb.;5(2): 164–78.

Chang, J. 2017. Texas Medical Board Sanctions Controversial Cancer Doctor Burzynski. *Austin-Statesman*, Mar. 3. http://www.mystatesman.com/news

/texas-medical-board-sanctions-controversial-cancer-doctor-burzynski /L9lDsfNTbBOuaWWqLEDBUI/, acc. Oct. 28, 2017.

Chen, C, & D Burger. 2015. Sarepta CEO Quits; Successor Pledges to Work Better with FDA. *Bloomberg Business*, Mar. 31. http://www.bloomberg.com/news /articles/2015-04-01/duchenne-biotech-firm-sarepta-s-ceo-chris-garabedian -resigns, acc. Aug. 7, 2016.

Christopher, WL. 1993. Off-Label Drug Prescription: Filling the Regulatory Vacuum. *Food and Drug Law Journal,* 48(2): 247–62.

Cimons, M. 1987. US Approves Sale of AZT to AIDS Patients. *Los Angeles Times*, Mar. 21. http://articles.latimes.com/1987-03-21/news/mn-4526_1_other-aids -patients, acc. May 26, 2016.

Cirak, S, V Arechavala-Gomeza, M Guglieri, et al. 2011. Exon Skipping and Dystrophin Restoration in Patients with Duchenne Muscular Dystrophy after Systemic Phosphorodiamidate Morpholino Oligomer Treatment: An Open-Label, Phase 2, Dose-Escalation Study. *Lancet,* Aug. 13; 378(9791): 595–605.

Clymer, HA. 1970. The Changing Costs and Risks of Pharmaceutical Innovation. In *The Economics of Drug Innovation*, ed. JD Cooper. (Washington, DC: American University), 123–24.

CNN. 2005. Journal Releases Vioxx Study. CNN.com Jan. 25. http://www.cnn .com/2005/health/01/25/vioxx.study.ap/, acc. May 22, 2012.

Competitive Enterprise Institute. 1995. A National Survey of Oncologists Regarding the Food and Drug Administration (August), Washington, DC.

———. 1996. A National Survey of Cardiologists Regarding the Food and Drug Administration. July. Washington, DC.

Conko, G. 2011. Hidden Truth: The Perils and Protection of Off-Label Drug and Medical Device Promotion. *Health Matrix*, 21: 149–87, esp. 154.

Conner, S. 2003. Glaxo Chief: Our Drugs Do Not Work on Most Patients. Dec. 8. http://www.independent.co.uk/news/science/glaxo-chief-our-drugs-do-not -work-on-most-patients-5508670.html, acc. Nov. 5, 2017.

ConsumerLab.com. n.d. Homepage. https://www.consumerlab.com/, acc. Nov. 5, 2017.

Cooper, JD, ed. 1970. *The Economics of Drug Innovation*. (Washington, DC: American University).

Crouch, G. 1991. Maker of AIDS Drug Accused of Securities Fraud: Pharmaceuticals: ICN of Costa Mesa and a Subsidiary Were Sued by the SEC for Misleading the Public about Ribavirin. Without Admitting Wrongdoing, They Signed

a Decree Not to Violate Statutes. *Los Angeles Times*, Oct. 8. http://articles.la
times.com/1991-10-08/business/fi-82_1_securities-fraud, acc. Sep. 24, 2017.

Cutler, D, M McClellan, & J Newhouse. 1997. The Costs and Benefits of Intensive Treatment for Cardiovascular Disease. Paper presented at American Enterprise Institute/Brookings Institution Conference on Measuring the Prices of Medical Treatments, Dec.

Czeizel, D. 1992. Prevention of the First Occurrence of Neural-Tube Defects by Periconceptional Vitamin Supplementation. *New England Journal of Medicine* Dec. 24;327(26): 1832–35.

De Walle, HEK, LTW De Jong-Van den Berg, & MC Cornel. 1999. Periconceptional Folic Acid Intake in the Northern Netherlands. *Lancet*, Apr. 3;353(9159): 1187.

De Walle, HEK, KM Van der Pal, LTW De Jong–Van den Berg, et al. 1998 Periconceptional Folic Acid in the Netherlands in 1995: Socioeconomic Differences. *Journal of Epidemiology and Community Health*, Dec.;52(12): 826–27.

Diamond, D. 2017. Lawmakers Defend "Unprecedented" Pentagon Health Panel, Which Could Undermine FDA: FDA Currently Has Sole Authority to Authorize Drugs and Devices for Emergency Use. Nov. 6. https://www.politico.com/story/2017/11/06/defense-department-health-committee-fda-drugs-military-244604, acc. Nov. 11, 2017.

DiMasi, JA. 2001a. New Drug Development in the United States from 1963 to 1999. *Clinical Pharmacology and Therapeutics,* May;69(5): 286–96, Figure 5.

———. 2001b. Risks in New Drug Development: Approval Success Rates for Investigational Drugs. *Clinical Pharmacology and Therapeutics*, May;69(5): 297–307, Tables I and Table II.

———. 2015. Regulation and Economics of Drug Development. Video presentation at the American Diabetes Association 75th Scientific Sessions, Boston, June 5. http://webcasts.diabetes.org/netadmin/Preview_redirect.aspx?lid=38132, acc. May 1, 2016.

DiMasi, JA, JS Brown, & L Lasagna. 1996. An Analysis of Regulatory Review Times of Supplemental Indications for Already-Approved Drugs: 1989–1994. *Therapeutic Innovation and Regulatory Science*, Apr. 30(2): 315–37.

DiMasi, JA, & HG Grabowski. 2007. The Cost of Biopharmaceutical R&D: Is Biotech Different? *Managerial and Decision Economics*, June;28: 469–79.

DiMasi, JA, HG Grabowski, & RW Hansen. 2016. Innovation in the Pharmaceutical Industry: New Estimates of R&D Costs. *Journal of Health Economics*, May;47: 20–33.

DiMasi, JA, RW Hansen, & HG Grabowski. 2003.The Price of Innovation: New Estimates of Drug Development Costs. *Journal of Health Economics*, Mar.;22(2): 151–85.

———. 2004. Assessing Claims about the Cost of New Drug Development: A Critique of the Public Citizen and TB Alliance Reports. http://csdd.tufts.edu /files/uploads/assessing_claims.pdf, acc. Nov. 18, 2013.

———. 2008. Misleading Congress about Drug Development: Reply. *Journal of Health Politics, Policy, and Law*, Apr.;33(2): 319–24; discussion 325–27.

DiMasi, JA, RW Hansen, HG Grabowski, et al. 1991. Cost of Innovation in the Pharmaceutical Industry. *Journal of Health Economics*;10: 107–42.

DiMasi, JA, JM Reichert, L Feldman, et al. 2013. Clinical Approval Success Rates for Investigational Cancer Drugs. *Clinical Pharmacology and Therapeutics*, Sep.;94(3): 329–35.

Dowling, HF. 1970. The American Medical Association's Policy on Drugs in Recent Decades. In *Safeguarding the Public: Historical Aspects of Medicinal Drug Control*, ed. JB Blake. (Baltimore, MD: Johns Hopkins University Press), 123–24.

Drug Watch. n.d. Androgel. http://www.drugwatch.com/testosterone/androgel/, acc. Dec. 10, 2015.

———. 2016. Vioxx Lawsuits: Claims Regarding Heart Attacks, Strokes, and Death. May. https://www.drugwatch.com/vioxx/lawsuit/, acc. Feb. 3, 2017.

Eli Lilly Company. 1972. The Lilly Digest. (Indianapolis, IN: Eli Lilly Company), 24.

Elias, TD. 1996. Doctor's Lifesaving Effort Could Land Him in Prison: FDA Ignores Cancer Drug's Success. *Washington Times*, Dec. 5.

Emord, JW. 2006. FDA Violation of the Rule of Law (1). Presented Sep. 23 at the Health Freedom Expo in Richmond, VA. http://www.emord.com/Read-FDA-Violation-of-the-Rule-of-Law.html, acc. on Jan. 12, 2014.

———. 2013 The Uncoupling of Injury from Adulteration. Jan. 11. http://emord .com/blawg/the-uncoupling-of-injury-from-adulteration/, acc. Jan. 29, 2017.

Epstein, RA. 2013. The FDA's Misguided Regulation of Stem-Cell Procedures: How Administrative Overreach Blocks Medical Innovation. *Legal Policy Report*, Sep.;17. https://www.manhattan-institute.org/pdf/lpr_17.pdf, acc. Oct. 31, 2017.

Faloon, W. 2004. As We See It: Cardiologists Overlook Lifesaving Discovery. *Life Extension Magazine*, Feb. http://www.lifeextension.com/magazine/2004/2 /awsi/page-01, acc. Oct. 11, 2015.

————. 2011. Pharmocarcy: How Corrupt Deals and Misguided Medical Regulations Are Bankrupting America—and What to Do About It. (Mount Jackson, VA: Praktikos Books), 7, 13, 79–80; 139, 204.

————. 2015. As We See It: CoQ10 Wars. *Life Extension Magazine*, Apr., 7–15, esp. 12–13.

————. 2017. As We See It: Unsustainable Drug Prices. *Life Extension Magazine*, Mar., 7–12, esp. 9.

Fang, MC, MC Perraillon, K Ghosh, et al. 2014. Trends in Stroke Rates, Risk, and Outcomes in the United States, 1988 to 2008. *American Journal of Medicine*, Jul.;127(7): 608–15.

Federal Register. 1969. 34 Fed Reg 14596 (Sep. 19), 130.12 (a)(5) and (7)(b)(iii).

Fein, AJ. 2014. Retail Generic Drug Inflation Reaches New Heights, Drug Channels. Aug. 12. http://www.drugchannels.net/2014/08/retail-generic-drug-inflation -reaches.html, acc. Mar. 22, 2015.

Fischl, A, DD Richman, MH Grieco, et al. 1987. The Efficacy of Azidothymidine (AZT) in the Treatment of Patients with AIDS and AIDS-related Complex. A Double-Blind, Placebo-Controlled Trial. *New England Journal of Medicine*, July 23;317(4): 185–91.

FitzGerald, GA. 2003. COX-2 and Beyond: Approaches to Prostaglandin Inhibition in Human Disease. *Nature Reviews/ Drug Discovery*, Nov.;2(11): 879–90.

————. 2004. Coxibs and Cardiovascular Disease. *New England Journal of Medicine*, Oct 21;351(17): 1709–11.

————. 2000. One-Year Follow-up of Patients Treated with Misoprostol in Acute Phase of Viral Hepatitis B. *Prostaglandins and Other Lipid Mediators*, Mar.;60(4-6).

Flisiak, R, & D Prokopowicz. 1997. Effect of Misoprostol on the Course of Viral Hepatitis B. *Hepatogastroenterology*, Sep.–Oct.;44(17): 1419–25.

————. 2000. One Year Follow-up of Patients Treated with Misoprostol in Acute Phase of Viral Hepatitis B. *Prostaglandins and Other Lipid Mediators*, Mar;60(4-6): 161–65.

Forbes. 2015. Why Are Generic Drug Prices Shooting Up? *Forbes*, Feb. 27. http:// www.forbes.com/sites/greatspeculations/2015/02/27/why-are-generic-drug -prices-shooting-up/print/, acc. Mar. 22, 2016.

Foulkes, AE. 2004. Weakened Immunity How the Food and Drug Administration Caused Recent Vaccine-Supply Problems. *Independent Review Summer*, Jan.;9(1): 31–54.

Furmark, T, L Appel, S Henningsson, et al. 2008. A Link Between Serotonin-Re-
lated Gene Polymorphisms, Amygdala Activity, and Placebo-Induced Relief
from Social Anxiety. *Journal of Neuroscience*, Dec. 3;28(49): 13066–743.

Gallo, RC, SZ Salahuddin, M Popovic, et al., 1984. Frequent Detection and Isolation of Cytopathic Retroviruses (HTLV-III) from Patients with AIDS and at
Risk for AIDS. *Science*, May 4;224(4648): 500–03.

Ganji, V, X Zhang, & V Tangpricha. 2012. Serum 25-HydroxyVitamin D Concentrations and Prevalence Estimates of Hypovitaminosis D in the US Population
Based on Assay-Adjusted Data. *Journal of Nutrition*, Mar.;142(3): 498–507.

Garrison, O. 1970. The Dictocrats. (New York: ARC Books), 75.

Georgiou, T, A Neokleous, D Nicolaou, et al. 2014. Pilot Study for Treating Dry
Age-Related Macular Degeneration (AMD) with High-Dose Omega-3 Fatty
Acids. *PharmaNutrition*, Jan.;2(1): 8–11.

Georgiou, T, & E Prokopiou. 2015. The New Era of Omega-3 Fatty Acids Supplementation: Therapeutic Effects on Dry Age-Related Macular Degeneration.
Journal of Stem Cells, I;10(3): 205–15.

Gerstenblith, AT, DE Baskin, CP Shah, et al. 2013. Electroretinographic Effects
of Omega 3 Fatty Acid Supplementation on Dry Age Related Macular Degeneration. *Journal of the American Medical Association of Ophthalmology*,
Mar.;131(3): 365–69.

Getz, KA, & KI Kaitin. 2015. Why Is the Pharmaceutical Industry Struggling? In
Re-Engineering Clinical Trials, eds. P Schuber and BM Buckley. (London: Academic Press), 3–15.

Gieringer, DH. 1985. The Safety and Efficacy of New Drug Approval. *Cato Journal*,
Spring/Summer;5(1): 177–201, esp. 185–87.

Gilbert, J, P Henske, & A Singh. 2003. Rebuilding Big Pharma's Business Model. *In
Vivo: The Business and Medical Report*;21(10): 1–10.

Giovannucci, E, Y Liu, BW Hollis, et al. 2008. Prospective Study of 25-Hydroxy-Vi-
tamin D and Risk of Myocardial Infarction in Men. *Archives of Internal Medicine*, June 9;168(11): 1174–80.

Global Alliance for TB Drug Development. 2001.The Economics of TB Drug Development. Oct. White paper, Global Alliance, New York.

Goldberg, R. 1997. David Kessler's Legacy at the FDA. Institute for Policy Innovation
Policy Report #143. http://www.ipi.org/docLib/QS143FDA.pdf-OpenElement
.pdf, acc. Sep. 11, 2017.

GoldenbergLaw PLLC. n.d. Overview of Vioxx Litigation. http://www.goldenber-
glaw.com/Vioxx-Litigation-Overview.html, acc. Feb. 2, 2017.

Goldman, DP, Y Zheng, F Girosi, et al. 2009. The Benefits of Risk Factor Prevention in Americans Aged 51 Years and Older. *American Journal of Public Health*, Nov.; 99(11): 2096–101.

Goldstein, LA, JS. Edelstein, & M Roth. 2012. Diamond Foods Settles Suit over Walnut Claims. Manatt Phelps and Phillips LLP. Jan. 20. https://www.lexology.com/library/detail.aspx?g=154c440d-cf31-405b-8ed1-e4aaae919279, acc. Nov. 3, 2017.

Goldwater Institute. 2016. Texas Right to Try Law Being Used to Successfully Treat Cancer Patients. Sep. 22. http://www.goldwaterinstitute.org/en/work/topics/healthcare/right-to-try/texas-right-to-try-law-being-used-to-successfully-/, acc. Jan. 14, 2017.

———. 2017. Pennsylvania Becomes 38th State to Pass Right to Try. Oct. 1. http://goldwaterinstitute.org/article/pennsylvania-becomes-38th-state-to-pass-right-to-try/, acc. Nov. 5, 2017.

Gonzalez-Gross, M, J Valtuena, C Breidenassel, et al. 2012. Vitamin D Status among Adolescents in Europe: The Healthy Lifestyle in Europe by Nutrition in Adolescence Study. *British Journal of Nutrition*, Mar.;107(5): 755–64.

Danaei, G, EL Ding, D Mozaffarian, et al. 2009. The Preventable Causes of Death in the United States: Comparative Risk Assessment of Dietary, Lifestyle, and Metabolic Risk Factors. *PLOS Medicine*, Apr. 6(4): e1000058. https://doi.org/10.1371/journal.pmed.1000058, acc. Jan. 22, 2018.

Graber, C. 2007. Snake Oil Salesmen Were on to Something: Snake Oil Really Is a Cure for What Ails You, If That Happens to Be Arthritis, Heart Disease, or Maybe Even Depression. *Scientific American*, Nov. 1. https://www.scientificamerican.com/article/snake-oil-salesmen-knew-something/, acc. Nov. 5, 2017.

Graham, DJ. 2004. Testimony, Nov. 18. https://www.finance.senate.gov/imo/media/doc/111804dgtest.pdf, acc. Oct. 31, 2107.

Grabowski, HG. 1976. Drug Regulation and Innovation: Empirical Evidence and Policy. (Washington, DC: American Enterprise Institute), 27, 37, 57, 60.

———. 1980. Regulation and the International Diffusion of Pharmaceuticals. In *The International Supply of Medicines*, ed. RB Helms. (Washington, DC: American Enterprise Institute), 5–36.

Grabowski, HG, J Vernon, & JA DiMasi. 2002. Returns on Research and Development for 1990s New Drug Introductions. *Pharmacoeconomica*;20 Suppl. 3: 11–29, esp. 22–23.

Grabowski, HG, JM Vernon, & LG Thomas. 1978. Estimating the Effects of Regulation on Innovation: An International Comparative Analysis of the Pharmaceutical Industry. *Journal of Law, Economics, and Policy*, Apr.; 21(1): 133–63, esp. 144–45.

Graham, DJ, D Campen, R Hui, et al. 2005. Risk of Acute Myocardial Infarction and Sudden Cardiac Death in Patients Treated with Cyclo-Oxygenase 2 Selective and Non-Selective Non-Steroidal Anti-Inflammatory Drugs: Nested Case-Control Study. *Lancet*, Feb. 5–11;365(9458): 475–81.

Grant, WB. 2009. In Defense of the Sun: An Estimate of Changes in Mortality Rates in the United States If Mean Serum 25-Hydroxyvitamin D Levels Were Raised to 45 ng/mL by Solar Ultraviolet-B Irradiance. *Dermato-Endocrinology*, July;1(4): 207–14.

———. 2011. An Estimate of the Global Reduction in Mortality Rates through Doubling Vitamin D Levels. *European Journal of Clinical Nutrition*, Sep.;65(9): 1016–26.

Greene-Finestone, LS, C Berger, M de Groh, et al. 2011. 25-Hydroxyvitamin D in Canadian Adults: Biological, Environmental, and Behavioral Correlates. *Osteoporosis International*, May;22(5): 1389–99.

Greig, PD, R Cameron, MJ Phillips, et al. 1994. Prostaglandin E in the Treatment of Recurrent Hepatitis B Infection after Orthotropic Liver Transplantation. *Transplantation*, July 27;58(2): 183–92.

Grow, JA. 1997. The Legislative History of the 1962 Amendments: A Failure to Forget or a Lesson to Learn From? *Harvard Law School Written Work Requirement*, May 1, 4.

Gruppo Italiano per lo Studio della Sopravvivenza Nell'Infarto Miocardico. 1999. Dietary Supplementation with N-3 Polyunsaturated Fatty Acids and Vitamin E after Myocardial Infarction: Results of the GISSI-Prevenzione Trial. *Lancet*, Aug. 7;354(9177): 447–55.

Hanley, R. 1986. Isoprinosine Maker Fights for FDA's OK. *Los Angeles Times*, Sep. 21. http://articles.latimes.com/1986-09-21/business/fi-9016_1_fda-approval, acc. May 23, 2016.

Hansen, RW. 1979. The Pharmaceutical Development Process: Estimates of Current Development Times and Effects of Regulatory Changes. In *Issues in Pharmaceutical Economics*, ed. RI Chien. (Lexington, MA: Lexington Books), 166.

Harris, G. 2009. Where Cancer Progress Is Rare, One Man Says No. *New York Times*, Sep. 15. http://www.nytimes.com/2009/09/16/health/policy/16cancer. html, acc. Jan.14, 2017.

———.2016. F.D.A. Regulator, Widowed by Cancer, Helps Speed Drug Approval. Jan. 2. https://www.nytimes.com/2016/01/03/us/politics/fda-regulator-widowed -by-cancer-helps-speed-drug-approval.html?_r=0, acc. Jan.14, 2017.

Hay, H, DW Thomas, JL Craighead, et al. 2014. Clinical Development Success Rates for Investigational Drugs. *Nature Biotechnology*, Jan.;32(1): 40–51.

Heaton, CA. 1994. The Chemical Industry. (Dordrecht, Netherlands: Springer), 40.

Heidenreich, P, & MB McClellan. 2001.Trends in Heart Attack Treatment and Outcomes, 1975–1995—Literature Review and Synthesis. In *Medical Care Output and Productivity*, eds. DM Cutler and ER Berndt. (Chicago: University of Chicago Press, 2001), 363–410, Table 9.2

Helfand, C. 2016a. FDA Swats Down T's EpiPen Copy, Putting Mylan in Cruise Control. *Fierce Pharma*, Mar. 1. http://www.fiercepharma.com/sales-and -marketing/fda-swats-down-teva-s-epipen-copy-putting-mylan-cruise -control, acc. Sep. 18, 2017.

———. 2016b. Curses, EpiPen! Another Would-Be Rival Falls Flat at FDA, Leaving Mylan's Med Unchallenged. *Fierce Pharma*, June 9. http://www.fiercepharma .com/marketing/still-no-epipen-challenge-sight-for-mylan-as-another -competitor-hits-a-snag, acc. Sep. 18, 2017.

Hemming, AW, MS Cattral, PD Greig, et al. 1996. The University of Toronto Liver Transplant Program. *Clinical Transplants,* 177–85.

Herrell, WE. 1943. Further Observations on the Clinical Use of Penicillin. *Proceedings of the Staff Meetings. Mayo Clinic*, 18: 65–76, esp. 71.

Higgs, R. 1994. An FDA Fable. *Reason Magazine*, Oct. https://reason.com /archives/1994/10/01/an-fda-fable, acc. Feb. 8, 2016.

Holick, MF. 2005. The Vitamin D Epidemic and Its Health Consequences. *Journal of* Nutrition, Nov.;135(11): 2739S–48S.

Horwitz, JP, J Chua, & MJ Noe. 1964. The Monomesylates of 1-(2-Deoxy-bd-Lyx-ofuranosyl)thymines. *Organic Chemistry Series Monographs*;29(7): 2076–79.

Hough, C. n.d. Photograph. https://commons.wikimedia.org/wiki/File:Unicap_ Upjohn.jpg, acc. Oct 31, 2017.

Howard, RL, AJ Avery, S Slavenburg, & S Royal. 2007. Which Drugs Cause Preventable Admissions to Hospital? A Systematic Review. *British Journal of Clinical Pharmacology*, Feb.; 63(2): 136–47.

Huber, PW. 2013. The Cure in the Code: How 20th Century Law Is Undermining 21st Century Medicine. (Philadelphia, PA: Basic Books).

Hyman, A, C Yim, M Krajden, et al. 1999. Oral Prostaglandin (PGE2) Therapy for Chronic Viral Hepatitis B and C. *Journal of Viral Hepatitis*, July;6(4): 329–36.

Hypponen, E, E Laara, A Reunanen, et al. 2001. Intake of Vitamin D and Risk of Type 1 Diabetes: A Birth Cohort Study. *Lancet*, Nov. 3;358(9292).

Idlebrook, C. 2014. Insulin Allergies Are for Real: Modern Formulas of Insulin Have Helped Curb Allergy Reactions, but Not Eliminated Them. June 24. http://insulinnation.com/treatment/medicine-drugs/insulin-allergies-are-for-real/, acc. May 29, 2016.

Institute for Safe Medication Practices. 2012. Anticoagulants the Leading Reported Drug Risk in 2011. *QuarterWatch*, May 31. https://www.ismp.org/quarterwatch/pdfs/2011Q4.pdf, acc. Nov. 12, 2017.

Jackson, CO. 1970. Food and Drug Legislation in the New Deal. (Princeton, NJ: Princeton University Press), 17–22.

Jadrow, JM. 1970. The Economic Effects of the 1962 Drug Amendments [dissertation]. (Charlottesville: University of Virginia), 38, 158, 160–61, 175–88.

Jaffe, R. 2016. FDA Draft Stem Cell Guidance Documents Exposed as Improper Rulemaking. *Bad Science and Heartless Public Policy*, Sep. 13, 2016. http://rickjaffeesq.com/2016/09/13/fda-draft-stem-cell-guidance-documents-exposed-improper-rulemaking-bad-science-heartless-public-policy/, acc. Oct. 2, 2016.

Jain, MK, & PM Ridker. 2005. Anti-Inflammatory Effects of Statins: Clinical Evidence and Basic Mechanisms, Nature Reviews. *Drug Discovery*, Dec.;4(12): 977–87.

Jenkins, HW Jr. 2001. Of Germs and Geopolitics. *Wall Street Journal*, Oct. 24, A23.

Jondrow, JA. 1972. Measure of the Monetary Benefits and Costs to Consumers of the Regulation of Prescription Drug Effectiveness [dissertation]. (Madison: University of Wisconsin), 15–16, 21–22, 27–29, 70, 72–73, 87–89, 109–10.

Kaitin, KI, & JS Brown. A Drug Lag Update. *Drug Information Journal*, 1995;29(2): 361–73.

Kaitin, KI, & C Cairns. 2003. The New Drug Approvals of 1999, 2000, and 2001: Drug Development Trends a Decade after Passage of the Prescription Drug User Fee Act of 1992. *Drug Information Journal*, Oct.;37(4): 357–71.

Kaitin, KI, N Mattison, FK Northington, et al. 1989. The Drug Lag: An Update of New Introductions in the United States and in the United Kingdom, 1977 through 1987. *Clinical Pharmacology and Therapeutics*, Aug;46(2): 121–38.

Kaplan, AH. 1995. Fifty Years of Drug Amendments Revisited: In Easy-to-Swallow Capsule Form. *Food and Drug Law Journal*, 50(Spec): 179–96, esp. 195.

Kazman, S. 1991. The FDA's Deadly Approval Process. *Consumers' Research*, Apr., 31.

Kennedy, B. 2013. The Pyridoxamine Trap. Jan. 11. http://emord.com/blawg/the-pyridoxamine-trap/, acc. Jan. 29, 2017.

Kent, S. 1994. A Pattern of Unlawful Behavior, FDA Raid Report: An Insider's Guide to Illegal and Unconstitutional Acts by the FDA. Dec. 1;2.

———. 1996. Victory over the FDA. *Life Extension Magazine*, Sep. http://www.lifeextension.com/magazine/1996/9/freedom/page-01, acc. Nov. 3, 2017.

Kirby, TJ Jr. 1962. Cataracts as Possible Complications of Treatment with Triparanol. *Archives of Ophthalmology*, Apr.; 67: 543–44.

KnowYourDose.org. 2017. Common Medicines. http://www.knowyourdose.org/common-medicines/, acc. Nov. 5, 2017.

Kolata, G. 1991. Patients Turning to Illegal Pharmacies. *New York Times*, Nov. 4, A1.

Kolberg, R. 1989. Generic Drug Scandal Widens. *United Press International*, July 11. http://www.upi.com/Archives/1989/07/11/Generic-drug-scandal-widens/2064616132800/, acc. Feb. 9, 2016.

Kovach, S. 2007. The Abigail Alliance Motivated by Tragic Circumstances, Families Battle an Uncaring Bureaucracy. *Life Extension Special Edition*. http://abigail-alliance.org/LEMSEP07pAbigailLR.pdf, acc. May 15, 2013.

Kvasz, M, IE Allen, MJ Gordon, et al. 2000. Adverse Drug Reactions in Hospitalized Patients: A Critique of a Meta-analysis. *Medscape General Medicine*, 2(2): published online. http://www.medscape.com/viewarticle/408052, acc. July 16, 2016.

Kwekkeboom, DJ, BL Kam, M Van Essen, et al. 2010. Somatostatin-Receptor-Based Imaging and Therapy of Gastroenteropancreatic Neuroendocrine Tumors. *Endocrine Related Cancer*, Jan. 29;17(1): R53–73.

Kwitny, J. 1992. Acceptable Risks. (New York: Poseidon Press), 78, 101–03, 146–47, 155–60, 167, 181–84, 187, 349–50, 423–24.

LaMattina, JL. 2011. Drug Truths: Why Should Wall Street Dictate the Level of Pharma R&D Spending? https://johnlamattina.wordpress.com/2011/10/18/why-should-wall-street-dictate-the-level-of-pharma-rd-spending/, acc. Sep. 11, 2016.

———. 2013. Devalued and Distrusted: Can the Pharmaceutical Industry Restore Its Broken Image? (Hoboken, NJ: John Wiley & Sons), 27–29, 32–37, 66, 71, 110–12.

LaRosa, JC, J He, & V Sjama. 1999. Effect of Statins on Risk of Coronary Disease: A Meta-Analysis of Randomized Controlled Trials. *Journal of the American Medical Association*, Dec. 22–29;282(24): 2340–46.

Larson, E. 1992. Unequal Treatments. *Reason Magazine*, Apr.; 48–50. https://reason.com/archives/1992/04/01/unequal-treatments, acc. Jan. 8, 2018.

Lasagna, L. 1989. Congress, the FDA, and New Drug Development: Before and After 1962. *Perspectives in Biology and Medicine*, Spring;32(3): 322–34.

Lasagna, L, & WM Wardell. 1975. The Rate of New Drug Discovery. In *Drug Development and Marketing*, ed. RB Helms. (Washington, DC: American Enterprise Institute for Public Policy Research): 157.

Laughlin, RC, & TF Carey. 1962. Cataracts in Patients Treated with Triparanol. *Journal of the American Medical Association*, July 28;181: 339–40.

Lazarou, J, BH Pomeranz, & PN Corey. 1998. Incidence of Adverse Drug Reactions in Hospitalized Patients. *Journal of the American Medical Association*, Apr. 15;279(15): 1200–05.

Lee, WM. 2004. Acetaminophen and the US Acute Liver Failure Study Group: Lowering the Risks of Hepatic Failure. Hepatology, July;40(1): 6–9.

Lichtenberg, FR. 1996. Do (More and Better) Drugs Keep People Out of Hospitals? *American Economic Review*, May;86(2): 384–88.

———. 2002. Sources of US Longevity Increase, 1960–1997. *NBER Working Paper* #w8755. http://www.nber.org/papers/w8755.pdf, acc. Jan. 8, 2018.

———. 2003a. Pharmaceutical Innovation, Mortality Reduction, and Economic Growth. In *Measuring the Gains from Medical Research: An Economic Approach*, eds. KM Murphy and RH Topel. (Chicago: University of Chicago Press), 74–109.

———. 2003b. The Benefits of Society to New Drugs: A Survey of the Econometric Evidence. *Proceedings of the Federal Reserve Bank of Dallas*, Sep. 43–59.

———. 2007. Benefits and Costs of New Drugs: An Update. *Managerial and Decision Economics*, June–Aug.;28(4-5): 485–90.

Lichtenberg, FR, & S Virabhak. 2007. Pharmaceutical-Embodied Technical Progress, Longevity, and Quality of Life: Drugs as Equipment for Your Health. *Managerial and Decision Economics*;28(4-5): 371–92.

LifeExtension. n.d. Homepage. http://www.lef.org, acc. Nov. 11, 2014.

Life Extension Foundation (LEF). 1994. *Life Extension Report*. Nov.;14(11):86.

———. 1995. The FDA Threatens Criminal Charges Against Offshore Pharmacies, FDA Raid Report: The Insider's Guide to Illegal and Unconstitutional Acts by the FDA. (Fort Lauderdale, FL: Life Extension Foundation), 1–5.

———. 2010. FDA Failure, Deception, Abuse: The Story of an Out-of-Control Government Agency and What It Means for Your Health. (Mount Jackson, VA: Praktikos Books), 474.

———. 2017. Life Extension Track Record, An Impeccable Track Record of 37 Years of Scientific Achievements in Health and Longevity. http://www .lifeextension.com/About/Lef-Scientific-Achievements-In-Health-And -Longevity_01, acc. Jan. 9, 2018.

Lim, MJ, SR Kwon, S Lee, et al. 2006. Rapid Improvement of Distal Vasculitis in PAN Related to Hepatitis B with Alprostadil Infusion: A Case Report. *Rheumatology International*, Aug.;26(10): 928–32.

Lindenmayer, JM, S Schoenfeld, R O'Grady, et al. 1998. Methicillin-Resistant Staphylococcus Aureus in a High School Wrestling Team and the Surrounding Community. *Archives of Internal Medicine*, Apr. 27;158(8): 895–99.

Lindren, K. 1986. Drug Firm to Alter Claims for Ribavirin at FDA Order. *Los Angeles Times*, Apr. 14. http://articles.latimes.com/1986-04-14/local/me-3874 _1_fda-approval, acc. Sep. 24, 2017.

Litchfield, J. 1962. Evaluation of the Safety of New Drugs by Means of Tests in Animals. *Clinical Pharmacology and Therapeutics*, Sep.–Oct.;3: 665–72.

Liu, JJ, J Prescott, E Giovannucci, et al. 2013. Plasma Vitamin D Biomarkers and Leukocyte Telomere Length. *American Journal of Epidemiology*, June 15;177(12): 1411–17.

Liu, K, PF Bross, & C Whitten. 2007. Biologics License Application (BLA) Medical Review Submission Number: BLA125197, 05/2/07. http://www.fda.gov /downloads/BiologicsBloodVaccines/CellularGeneTherapyProducts /ApprovedProducts/UCM214560.pdf, acc. Dec. 19, 2015.

Lockwood, K, S Moesgaard, & K Folkers. 1994. Partial and Complete Regression of Breast Cancer in Patients in Relation to Dosage of Coenzyme Q10. *Biochemical and Biophysical Research Communications*, Mar. 30;199(3): 1504–08.

Lockwood, K, S Moesgaard, T Hanioka, et al. 1994. Apparent Partial Remission of Breast Cancer in "High Risk" Patients Supplemented with Nutritional Antioxidants, Essential Fatty Acids, and Coenzyme Q10. *Molecular Aspects of Medicine*, 15(suppl): S231–40.

Lockwood, K, S Moesgaard, T Yamamoto, et al. 1995. Progress on Therapy of Breast Cancer with Vitamin Q10 and the Regression of Metastases. *Biochemical and Biophysical Research Communications*, July 6;212(1): 172–77.

Loftus, P. 2016. Merck to Pay $830 Million to Settle Vioxx Shareholder Suit: Settlement Moves Drug Company Closer to Resolving Litigation Surrounding Pulled Painkiller. Jan. 15. https://www.wsj.com/articles/merck-to-pay-830 -million-to-settle-vioxx-shareholder-suit-1452866882, acc. Feb. 3, 2017.

Long, G, & J Works. 2013. *Innovation in the Biopharmaceutical Pipeline: A Multidimensional View.* (Boston: Analysis Group Inc.), 11.

Loudon, M. 2005. The FDA Exposed: An Interview with Dr. David Graham, the Vioxx Whistleblower. http://www.naturalnews.com/011401_Dr_David _Graham_the_FDA.html, acc. Dec. 29, 2013.

Lowe, D. 2011. Makena's Price: What to Do? *In the Pipeline,* Mar. 11. http://blogs. sciencemag.org/pipeline/archives/2011/03/11/makenas_price_what_to_do, acc. June 11, 2016.

———. 2014. The Most Unconscionable Drug Price Hike I Have Yet Seen. *In the Pipeline,* Sep. 11. http://blogs.sciencemag.org/pipeline/archives/2014/09/11 /the_most_unconscionable_drug_price_hike_i_have_yet_seen, acc. June 11, 2016.

———. 2015. M Shkreli Has One Idea and It's a Bad One. *In the Pipeline,* Sep. 21. http://blogs.sciencemag.org/pipeline/archives/2015/09/21/martin-shkreli -has-one-idea-and-its-a-bad-one, acc. Aug. 1, 2016.

Lucas, RM, AL Ponsonby, JA Pasco, et al. 2008. Future Health Implications of Prenatal and Early-Life Vitamin D Status. *Nutrition Reviews,* Dec.;66(12): 710–20.

Hypponen, E, E Laara, A Reunanen, et al. 2001. Intake of Vitamin D and Risk of Type 1 Diabetes: A Birth Cohort Study. *Lancet,* Nov. 3;358(9292): 1500–03.

Lynes, B. 1989. The Healing of Cancer. (Queensville, Ontario: Marcus Books), 22.

Lyytinen, H, E Pukkala, & O Ylikorkala. 2009. Breast Cancer Risk in Postmenopausal Women Using Estradiol-Progestogen Therapy. *Obstetrics and Gynecology,* Jan.;113(1): 65–73.

MacFarlane, N. n.d. The Secrets of Fish Oil Purity. http://docplayer.net/30502129- The-secrets-of-fish-oil-purity-neil-macfarlane-elloughton-hu151hp-england .html, acc. Feb. 6, 2017.

Maharrey, M. 2017. Signed by the Governor: Arizona Free Speech in Medicine Act Sets Stage to Nullify FDA Law. Mar. 24. http://blog.tenthamendmentcenter .com/2017/03/signed-by-the-governor-arizona-free-speech-in-medicine -act-sets-stage-to-nullify-fda-law/, acc. Apr. 15, 2017.

Mansfield, EH. 1970. "Discussion by Panel." In *The Economics of Drug Innovation,* ed. JD Cooper. (Washington, DC: American University).

Manzano, A, & P Pérez-Segura. 2012. Colorectal Cancer Chemoprevention: Is This the Future of Colorectal Cancer Prevention? *Scientific World Journal,* 327–41. doi: 10.1100/2012/327341.

Marcus, AD. 2012. Frustrated ALS Patients Concoct Their Own Drug. *Wall Street Journal,* Apr. 15. http://www.wsj.com/articles/SB10001424052702304818404 577345953943484054, acc. Sep. 4, 2017, and Oct. 31, 2017.

Matthews, AW, & B Martinez. 2004. Emails Suggest Merck Knew Vioxx's Dangers at Early Stage. *Wall Street Journal,* Nov. 1; A1.

May, MS, WM Wardell, & L Lasagna. 1983. New Drug Development During and After a Period of Regulatory Change: Clinical Research Activity of Major United States Pharmaceutical Firms, 1958–1979. *Clinical Pharmacology and Therapeutics,* June;33(6): 691–700.

Medical Letter. n.d. Homepage. http://secure.medicalletter.org/.

MedlinePlus. n.d. Duchenne Muscular Dystrophy. https://medlineplus.gov/ency /article/000705.htm, acc. Aug. 7, 2016.

Medtap International. n.d. The Value of Investment in Health Care: Better Care, Better Lives. p. 4. http://www.aha.org/content/00-10/Value_Report.pdf, acc. Oct. 28, 2017.

Mepact. n.d. Mepact: EPAR—Product Information. http://www.ema.europa. eu/docs/en_GB/document_library/EPAR_-_Product_Information/human /000802/WC500026565.pdf, acc. Feb. 9, 2016.

Meyler, L., ed. 1966. Side Effects of Drugs, Vol. V. (New York: Elsevier), 43–44.

Mihm, S. 2007. A Tragic Lesson. *Boston Globe,* Aug. 26. http://archive.boston.com /news/globe/ideas/articles/2007/08/26/a_tragic_lesson/, acc. Nov. 12, 2017.

Miller, HI. 2000. To America's Health: A Proposal to Reform the Food and Drug Administration. (Stanford, CA: Hoover Institution Press), 41–42.

Mills, EJ, P Wu, M Alberton, et al. 2012. Low-Dose Aspirin and Cancer Mortality: A Meta-Analysis of Randomized Trials. *American Journal of Medicine,* June;125(6): 560–67.

Milunsky, A, H Jick, SS Jick, et al. 1989. Multivitamin/Folic Acid Supplementation in Early Pregnancy Reduces the Prevalence of Neural Tube Defects. *Journal of the American Medical Association,* Nov. 24;262(20): 2847–52.

Mintz, M. 1969. FDA and Panalba: A Conflict of Commercial, Therapeutic Goals? *Science,* Aug. 29;165(3896): 875–81.

Mitsuya, H, M Popovic, R Yarchoan, et al. 1984. Suramin Protection of T Cells in Vitro against Infectivity and Cytopathic Effect of HTLV-III. *Science,* Oct. 12;226(4671): 172–74.

Mitsuya, H, KJ Weinhold, PA Furman, et al. 1985. 3'-Azido-3'-Deoxythymidine (BW A509U): An Antiviral Agent that Inhibits the Infectivity and Cytopathic Effect of Human T-Lymphotropic Virus Type III/Lymphadenopathy

Associated Virus in Vitro. *Proceedings of the National Academy of Sciences USA*;82: 7096–100.

Morand, GB, SD da Silva, MP Hier, et al. 2014. Insights into Genetic and Epigenetic Determinants with Impact on Vitamin D Signaling and Cancer Association Studies: The Case of Thyroid Cancer. *Frontiers in Oncology*, Nov. 4;4: 309.

Morgenthaler, J, & JV Wright. 1997. Natural Hormone Replacement for Women over 45. (Walnut, CA: Smart Publications).

Mortensen, SA, F Rosenfeldt, A Kumar, et al. 2014. The Effect of Coenzyme Q10 on Morbidity and Mortality in Chronic Heart Failure: Results from Q-SYM-BIO: A Randomized Double-Blind Trial. *JACC. Heart Failure*, Dec.;2(6): 641–49.

Mukherjee, D, SE Nissen, & EJ Topol. 2001. Risk of Cardiovascular Events Associated with Selective COX-2 Inhibitors. *Journal of the American Medical Association*, Aug. 22–29;286(8): 954–59.

Mund, VA. 1970. The Return on Investment of the Innovative Pharmaceutical Firm. In *The Economics of Drug Innovation*, ed. JD Cooper. (Washington, DC: American University), 125–38.

Munger, KL, SM Zhang, E O'Reilly, et al. 2004. Vitamin D Intake and Incidence of Multiple Sclerosis. *Neurology*, Jan. 13;62(1): 60–65.

Murphy, KM, & RH Topel. The Economic Value of Medical Research. In *Measuring the Gains from Medical Research: An Economic Approach*, eds KM Murphy & RH Toppel. (Chicago: University of Chicago Press, 2003), 41–73, esp. 42.

National Research Council (NRC). 1969. *Drug Efficacy Study: Final Report to the Commissioner of Food and Drugs, FDA*. (Washington, DC: National Academy of Sciences), 7, 12, 876.

Neuralstem Inc. 2016. Neuralstem Presented Cell Therapy Update at Phacilitate Cell and Gene Therapy World Conference, Jan. 27, 2016. https://investor. neuralstem.com/press-releases/detail/190/neuralstem-presented-cell-therapy-update-at-phacilitate, acc. Jan. 6, 2018.

Neuralstem Pipeline. n.d. About Amyotrophic Lateral Sclerosis (ALS). http://www.neuralstem.com/pipeline/ns-566, acc. Oct. 31, 2017.

New York Times. 1989. The Generic Drug Scandal. Oct. 2. http://www.nytimes .com/1989/10/02/opinion/the-generic-drug-scandal.html, acc. Mar. 30, 2017.

NCI Staff. 2017. Cancer Researchers Report Progress in Studying Exceptional Responders, July 6. https://www.cancer.gov/news-events/cancer-currents-blog /2017/exceptional-responders-progress, acc. Nov. 5, 2017.

Ng, K. 2014. Vitamin D for Prevention and Treatment of Colorectal Cancer: What is the Evidence? *Current Colorectal Cancer Reports*, Sep. 1;10(3): 339–45.

Nicholas, P. 1937. Elixir Sulfanilamide of Massengill Chemical: Chemical, Pharmacologic, Pathologic, and Necropsy Reports; Preliminary Toxicity Reports on Diethylene Glycol and Sulfanilamide. *Journal of the American Medical Association*, Nov. 6;109(19): 1531–39.

1918 Flu Pandemic. n.d. Wikipedia, note 3. http://en.wikipedia.org/wiki/1918 _flu_pandemic#cite_note-3, acc. Feb. 1, 2014.

Norton, R. 2001. Clinical Pharmacogenomics: Applications in Pharmaceutical R&D. *Drug Discovery Today*, Feb. 1;6(4): 180–85.

Offit, PA. 2005. The Cutter Incident: How America's First Polio Vaccine Led to the Growing Vaccine Crisis. (New Haven, CT: Yale University Press): 100, 116–19, 133.

Ogata, Y, K Matono, H Tsuda, et al. 2015. Randomized Phase II Study of 5-Fluorouracil Hepatic Arterial Infusion With or Without Antineoplastons as an Adjuvant Therapy after Hepatectomy for Liver Metastases from Colorectal Cancer. *PLoS One*, Mar. 19;10(3): published online.

O'Keefe, JH Jr., & WS Harris. 2000. From Inuit to Implementation: Omega-3 Fatty Acids Come of Age. *Mayo Clinic Proceedings*, June;75(6): 607–14.

Olsen, D. 2015. *The Right to Try: How the Federal Government Prevents Americans from Getting the Lifesaving Treatments They Need.* (New York: HarperCollins), 1–18, 37, 40, 59, 83–88.

Olson, MK. 2002. Pharmaceutical Policy Change and the Safety of New Drugs. *Journal of Law and Economics*, Oct.;45(S2): 615–31.

———. 2008. The Risk We Bear: The Effects of Review Speed and Industry User Fees on New Drug Safety. *Journal of Health and Economics*, Mar.;27(2): 175–200.

Orac. 2013. Stanislaw Burzynski in *USA Today*: Abuse of Clinical Trials and Patients Versus the Ineffectiveness of the FDA and Texas Medical Board. Nov. 15. http://scienceblogs.com/insolence/2013/11/15/stanislaw-burzynski-in-usa -today-abuse-of-clinical-trials-and-patients-versus-the-ineffectiveness-of -the-fda-and-texas-medical-board/, acc. Mar. 6, 2016.

Ostertag, W, G Roesler, CJ Krieg, et al. 1974. Induction of Endogenous Virus and of Thymidine Kinase by Bromodeoxyuridine in Cell Cultures Transformed by Friend Virus. *Proceedings of the National Academy of Sciences of the United States of America*, Dec.; 71(12): 4980–85.

Palca, J. 1992. Agencies Split on Nutrition Advice. *Science*, Sep. 25;257(5078): 1857.

Parfet, RT Jr. 1969. Upjohn's Position on Panalba, *Science*, Dec. 12;166(3911): 1354.

Patrycja, N, RA León de la Fuente, ST Nilsen, et al. 2013. Vitamin D Predicts All-Cause and Cardiac Mortality in Females with Suspected Acute Coronary Syndrome: A Comparison with Brain Natriuretic Peptide and High-Sensitivity C-Reactive Protein. *Cardiology Research and Practice*, 2013:398034. Epub Nov 17.

Patronas, N. 1993. Court Testimony, May 24. http://www.burzynskimovie.com /images/stories/Understanding/93_5_24_Patronas_Burzynski.pdf, acc. Oct. 31, 2017.

Paul, SM, DS Mytelka, CT Dunwiddie, et al. 2010. How to Improve R&D Productivity: The Pharmaceutical Industry's Grand Challenge. *Nature Reviews Drug Discovery*, 9: 203–14.

Pearson, D, & S Shaw. 1993. *Freedom of Informed Choice: FDA versus Nutrient Supplements*. (Neptune, NJ: Common Sense Press), 7.

Pedersen, C, E Sandstrom, CS Petersen, et al. 1990. The Efficacy of Inosine Pranobex in Preventing the Acquired Immunodeficiency Syndrome in Patients with Human Immunodeficiency Virus Infection. The Scandinavian Isoprinosine Study Group. *New England Journal of Medicine*, June 21;322(25): 1757–63.

Peltzman, S. 1973. An Evaluation of Consumer Protection Legislation: The 1962 Drug Amendments. *Journal of Political Economy*, Sep.–Oct.;81(5): 1049–91. Reformatted and colorized by FDAReview.org, a project of the Independent Institute reprinted with permission. http://www.fdareview.org/05_harm.php, acc. July 10, 2017.

———. 1974. *Regulation of Pharmaceutical Innovation: The 1962 Amendments*. (Washington, DC: American Enterprise Institute for Public Policy Research), 13–18, 53–54.

Petersen, M, & R Abelson. 2002. Drug Makers and F.D.A. Fighting Hard over Quality. *New York Times*, May 17. http://www.nytimes.com/2002/05/17/business /drug-makers-and-fda-fighting-hard-over-quality.html, acc. Feb. 21, 2014.

Pew Charitable Trusts. 2013. GAIN: How a New Law Is Stimulating the Development of Antibiotics. Nov. 7. http://www.pewtrusts.org/en/research-and-analysis /issue-briefs/2013/11/07/gain-how-a-new-law-is-stimulating-the-development -of-antibiotics, acc. May 21, 2016.

Pham, n.d. 2015. *IP Intensive Manufacturing Industries: Driving US Economic Growth*. (Washington, DC: NDP Analytics, Mar.), 13, Table 5, http://static1 .squarespace.com/static/52850a5ce4b068394a270176/t/5509888de4b05ef9d ed57e01/1426688141783/IP+Report+-+March+2015.pdf, acc. June 3, 2016.

Pharmaceutical Research and Manufacturers of America (PhRMA). 2012. *PhRMA 2012 Profile.* (Washington, DC: PhRMA), 30. http://www.phrma.org/sites/default/files/pdf/phrma_industry_profile.pdf, acc. May 9, 2013.

———. 2013. *2013 Biopharmaceutical Research Industry Profile.* (Washington, DC: PhRMA), ii.

———. 2015. *Biopharmaceutical Research Industry Profile.* (Washington, DC: PhRMA), 66.

———. 2016. *Chart Pack: Biopharmaceuticals in Perspective.* (Washington, DC: PhRMA), 110. http://phrma.org/sites/default/files/pdf/chart-pack-biopharmaceuticals-in-perspective.pdf, acc. June 3, 2016.

Pierce, JJ. 1995. Dangerous Excesses: A Look at the Food and Drug Administration. *Issue Analysis No. 13,* Citizens for a Sound Economy Foundation, Nov. 9.

Pittas, AG, B Dawson-Hughes, T Li, et al. 2006. Vitamin D and Calcium Intake in Relation to Type 2 Diabetes in Women. *Diabetes Care,* Mar;29(3): 650–56.

Pittas, AG, J Lau, F. Hu, et al. 2007. The Role of Vitamin D and Calcium in Type 2 Diabetes. A Systematic Review and Meta-Analysis. *Journal of Clinical Endocrinology and Metabolism,* June;92(6): 2007–29.

Pollack, A. 2015. Huge Hikes in Prices of Drugs Raise Protests and Questions. *New York Times,* Sep. 20. https://www.bostonglobe.com/business/2015/09/20/huge-overnight-increase-drug-price-raises-protests/DH94tAOlMzZVDIZj55Y6NP/story.html, acc. Aug. 1, 2016.

Pompidou, A, D Zagury, RC Gallo, et al. 1985. In-Vitro Inhibition of LAV/HTLV-III Infected Lymphocytes by Dithiocarb and Inosine Pranobex. *Lancet,* Dec. 21–28;2(8469-70): 1423.

Popovic, M, MG Sarngadharan, E Read, et al. 1984. Detection, Isolation, and Continuous Production of Cytopathic Retroviruses (HTLV-III) from Patients with AIDS and Pre-AIDS. *Science,* May 4;224(4648): 497–500.

Premkumar, VG, S Yuvaraj, K Vijayasarathy, et al. 2007. Effect of Coenzyme Q10, Riboflavin, and Niacin on Serum CEA and CA 15-3 Levels in Breast Cancer Patients Undergoing Tamoxifen Therapy. *Biological and Pharmaceutical Bulletin,* Feb.;30(2): 367–70.

Price, DD, DG Finniss, & F Benedetti. 2008. A Comprehensive Review of the Placebo Effect: Recent Advances and Current Thought. *Annual Review of Psychology,* 59: 565–90.

Public Citizen. 2001. Rx R&D Myths: The Case Against the Drug Industry's R&D Scare Card. http://www.citizen.org/documents/rdmyths.pdf, acc. Sep. 20, 2016.

Public Citizen's Health Research Group. 2011. Update on Withdrawals of Dangerous Drugs in the US. *Worst Pills, Best Pills Newsletter*, Jan. http://www.worstpills.org/includes/page.cfm?op_id=552#table1, acc. Oct. 21, 2007.

Public Law 97-414. 1983. The Orphan Drug Act. Jan. 4,. https://www.gpo.gov/fdsys/pkg/STATUTE-96/pdf/STATUTE-96-Pg2049.pdf, acc. Jan. 8, 2017.

Puri, RK. n.d. Development of Safe and Effective Tumor Vaccines and Gene Therapy Products. https://www.fda.gov/biologicsbloodvaccines/scienceresearch/biologicsresearchareas/ucm127167.htm, acc. June 4, 2017.

Quickwatch. 1998. The Antineoplaston Anomaly: How a Drug Was Used for Decades in Thousands of Patients, with No Safety, Efficacy Data. *The Cancer Letter*, Sep. 25; 24(36). https://www.quackwatch.org/01QuackeryRelatedTopics/Cancer/burzynski2.html, acc. Oct. 31, 2017.

Reus, S, M Priego, V Boix, et al. 1998. Can Alprostadil Improve Liver Failure in HIV-Infected Patients with Severe Acute Viral Hepatitis? *Journal of Infection*, July;37(1): 84–86.

Ricardo-Campbell, R. 1976. *Drug Lag: Federal Government Decision Making*. (Stanford, CA: Hoover Institution Press), 48.

Roan, S. 2007. Drug's Delay Mobilizes Prostate Patients to Activism. *Los Angeles Times*, Dec. 31.

Robert, A, PA Aristoff, MG Wendling, et al. 1985. Cytoprotective and Antisecretory Properties of a Non-Diarrheogenic and Non-Uterotonic Prostacyclin Analog: U-68,215. *Prostaglandins*, Oct.;30(4): 619–49.

Robert, A, JE Nezamis, C Lancaster, et al. 1979. Cytoprotection by Prostaglandins in Rats: Prevention of Gastric Necrosis Produced by Alcohol, HCl, NaOH, Hypertonic NaCl, and Thermal Injury. *Gastroenterology*, Sep.;77(3): 433–43.

Roberts, RB, GM Dickinson, PN Heseltine, et al. 1990. A Multicenter Clinical Trial of Oral Ribavirin in HIV-Infected Patients with Lymphadenopathy. The Ribavirin-LAS Collaborative Group. *Journal of Acquired Immune Deficiency Syndrome*, 3(9): 884–92.

Rosemann, A. 2014. Why Regenerative Stem Cell Medicine Progresses Slower Than Expected. *Journal of Cellular Biochemistry*, Dec.;115(12): 2073–76.

Ross, JS, D Madigan, KP Hill, et al. 2009. Pooled Analysis of Rofecoxib Placebo-Controlled Clinical Trial Data: Lessons for Post-Market Pharmaceutical Safety Surveillance. *Archives of Internal Medicine*, Nov. 23; 169(21): 1976–85.

Rothschild, NM. n.d. *Wikipedia*. http://en.wikipedia.org/wiki/Nathan_Mayer_Rothschild, acc. Dec. 7, 2013.

Rothwell, PM, JF Price, FGR Fowkes, et al. 2012. Short-Term Effects of Daily Aspirin on Cancer Incidence, Mortality, and Non-Vascular Death: Analysis of the Time Course of Risks and Benefits in 51 Randomized Controlled Trials. *Lancet*, 379(9826): 1602–12.

Rothwell, PM, M Wilson, CE Elwin, et al. 2010. Long-Term Effect of Aspirin on Colorectal Cancer Incidence and Mortality: 20-Year Follow-up of Five Randomized Trials. *Lancet*, Nov. 20;376(9754): 1741–50.

Rothwell, PM, M Wilson, JF Price, et al. 2012. Effect of Daily Aspirin on Risk of Cancer Metastasis: A Study of Incident Cancers during Randomized Controlled Trials. *Lancet*, 379 (9826): 1591–601.

Ruwart, MJ. 2004. Is Excess Regulation Responsible for Soaring Pharmaceutical Prices? American Association for Pharmaceutical Sciences Annual Meeting and Exposition, Nov. 7–11. http://abstracts.aaps.org/SecureView/AAPSJournal /radrezxgsa1.pdf, acc. Sep. 23, 2017.

———. 2005a. Cost-Benefit Estimates for the 1962 Kefauver-Harris Amendments. International Conference on Drug Development, Feb.

———. 2005b. Book Review: The $800 Million Pill: The Truth Behind the Cost of New Drugs, by M Goozner. *Journal of American Physicians and Surgeons*, Spring;10(1): 24.

———. 2015. *Healing Our World: The Compassion of Libertarianism*. (Kalamazoo, MI: SunStar Press), 67–82, chap. 7, 105–20, 53–150.

Sallmann, LV, P Grimes, & E Collins. 1963. Triparanol-Induced Cataract in Rats. *Transactions of the American Ophthalmology Society*, 61: 49–60, esp. 59.

Santo, J. 2015. Dendreon Gets Nod for Ch. 11 Liquidation Plan. *Law 360*, June 2. http://www.law360.com/articles/662623/dendreon-gets-nod-for-ch -11-liquidation-plan, acc. Mar. 27, 2016.

Sarepta. 2018. *Sarepta Therapeutics*. Our Pipeline. http://www.sarepta.com /our-pipeline, acc. Jan. 8, 2018.

Sarepta Therapeutics. 2012. Sarepta Therapeutics Announces Eteplirsen Meets Primary Endpoint of Increased Novel Dystrophin and Achieves Significant Clinical Benefit on 6-Minute Walk Test after 48 Weeks of Treatment in PhaseIIb Study in Duchenne Muscular Dystrophy. Oct. 3. http://www.marketwired .com/press-release/sarepta-therapeutics-announces-eteplirsen-meets -primary-endpoint-increased-novel-dystrophin-nasdaq-srpt-1708626.htm, acc. Nov. 5, 2017.

———. 2014. Sarepta Therapeutics Announces Eteplirsen Demonstrates Stability on Pulmonary Function Tests through 120 Weeks in Phase IIb Study in

Duchenne Muscular Dystrophy. Feb. 5. http://investorrelations.sarepta.com /news-releases/news-release-details/sarepta-therapeutics-announces -eteplirsen-demonstrates-stability, acc. Nov. 5, 2017.

———. 2017. Sarepta Therapeutics Announces Positive Results in Its Study Evaluating Gene Expression, Dystrophin Production, and Dystrophin Localization in Patients with Duchenne Muscular Dystrophy (DMD) Amenable to Skipping Exon 53 Treated with Golodirsen (SRP-4053). Sep. 6. https:// globenewswire.com/news-release/2017/09/06/1108211/0/en/Sarepta -Therapeutics-Announces-Positive-Results-in-Its-Study-Evaluating -Gene-Expression-Dystrophin-Production-and-Dystrophin-Localization -in-Patients-with-Duchenne-Muscular-Dystrop.html, acc. Nov. 5, 2017.

Sarett, LE. 1974. Impact of Regulation on Industrial R&D: FDA Regulations and Their Influence on Future R&D. *Research Management*, Mar.;17.

Sarngadharan, MG, M Popovic, L Bruch, et al. 1984. Antibodies Reactive with Human T-Lymphotropic Retroviruses (HTLV-III) in the Serum of Patients with AIDS. *Science*, May 4;224(4648): 506–08.

Schardein, JL. 1976. *Drugs as Tetrogens.* (Cleveland, OH: CRC Press), 5.

Schöttker, B, R Jorde, A Peasey, et al. 2014. Vitamin D and Mortality: Meta-Analysis of Individual Participant Data from a Large Consortium of Cohort Studies from Europe and the United States. *British Medical Journal*, June 17;348: g3656.

Schnee, JE. 1970. *Research and Technological Change in the Ethical Pharmaceutical Industry* [dissertation]. (Philadelphia: University of Pennsylvania), 220.

Schüpbach, J, M Popovic, RV Gilden, et al. 1984. Serological Analysis of a Subgroup of Human T-Lymphotropic RetroViruses (HTLV-III) Associated with AIDS. *Science*, May 4;224(4648): 503–05.

Schwartzman, D. 1975a. Pharmaceutical R&D Expenditures and Rates of Return. In *Drug Development and Marketing*, ed. RB Helms. (Washington, DC: American Enterprise Institute for Public Policy Research).

———. 1975b. *The Expected Return from Pharmaceutical Research.* (Washington, DC: American Enterprise Institute for Public Policy Research), 19.

———. 1976. *Innovation in the Pharmaceutical Industry.* (Baltimore, MD: John Hopkins University Press), 70.

Sears, B. 1995. *Enter the Zone: A Dietary Road Map.* (New York: ReganBooks).

Secure Medical Letter. n.d. The Medical Letter on Drugs and Therapeutics. (New Rochelle, NY: Medical Letter Inc.).

Sherman, W. 1992. Underground Medicine. *US News & World Report*, May 11, 62–69.

Shilts, R. 2007. *And the Band Played on: Politics, People, and the AIDS Epidemic.* (New York: St. Martin's Press).

Shorter, E. 1987. *The Health Century*. (New York: Doubleday), 68–70.

Shulman, R, JA DiMasi, & KI Kaitin. 1999. Patent Term Restoration: The Impact of the Waxman-Hatch Act on New Drugs and Biologics Approved 1984–1995. *Journal of BioLaw and Business*, 2: 63–68.

Silletta MG, LG Pioggiarella, G Levantesi, et al. 2009. Omega-3 Fatty Acids and Heart Failure. *Current Atherosclerosis Reports*, Nov.;11(6): 440–47.

Simon, KC, KL Munger, & A Ascherio. 2012. Vitamin D and Multiple Sclerosis: Epidemiology, Immunology, and Genetics. *Current Opinion in Neurology*, June;25(3): 246–51.

Sinclair, SB, PD Greig, LM Blendis, et al. 1989. Biochemical and Clinical Response of Fulminant Viral Hepatitis to Administration of Prostaglandin E. A Preliminary Report. *Journal of Clinical Investigation*, Oct.;84(4): 1063–69.

Sinclair, SB, & GA Levy. 1991. Treatment of Fulminant Viral Hepatic Failure with Prostaglandin E. A Preliminary Report. *Digestive Diseases and Science*, June;36(6): 791–800.

Singh, RB, NS Neki, K Kartikey, et al. 2003. Effect of Coenzyme Q10 on Risk of Atherosclerosis in Patients with Recent Myocardial Infarction. *Molecular and Cellular Biochemistry*, Apr.; 246(1–2): 75–82.

Sivanathan, N, & H Kakkar. 2017. The Unintended Consequences of Argument Dilution in Direct-to-Consumer Drug Advertisements. *Nature Human Behavior*, 1(10): 1–6.

Small, EJ, PF Schellhammer, CS Higano, et al. 2006. Placebo-Controlled Phase 1II Trial of Immunologic Therapy with Sipuleucel-T (APC8015) in Patients with Metastatic, Asymptomatic Hormone Refractory Prostate Cancer. *Journal of Clinical Oncology*, July 1;24(19): 3089–94.

Smart Patients. n.d. Dose-Ranging Study of AVI-4658 to Induce Dystrophin Expression in Selected Duchenne Muscular Dystrophy (DMD) Patients. https://www.smartpatients.com/trials/NCT00844597, acc. Aug. 7, 2016.

Smithells, RW, S Sheppard, CJ Schorah, et al. 1981. Apparent Prevention of Neural Tube Defects by Periconceptional Vitamin Supplements. *Archives of Disease in Childhood*, Dec.;56(12): 911–18.

Somers, S. 2011. Suzanne Somers' Stem Cell Breast Reconstruction Surgery. Uploaded Dec. 30. https://www.youtube.com/watch?v=xt55cTQEoHk&feature =youtu.be, acc. Oct. 2, 2016.

Somers, S, & RA Greene. 2005. *The Sexy Years: Discover the Hormone Connection: The Secret to Fabulous Sex, Great Health, and Vitality, for Women and Men.* (New York: Harmony Books).

Sonnedecker, G. 1970. Contribution of the Pharmaceutical Profession Toward Controlling the Quality of Drugs in the Nineteenth Century. In *Safeguarding the Public Health: Historical Aspects of Medicinal Drug Control,* ed. JB Blake. (Baltimore: Johns Hopkins University Press, 1970), 105–06.

Spedding, S, S Vanlint, H Morris, et al. 2013. Does Vitamin D Sufficiency Equate to a Single Serum 25-Hydroxyvitamin D Level or Are Different Levels Required for Non-Skeletal Diseases? *Nutrients,* Dec.;5(12): 5127–39.

Spellberg, B. 2009. *Rising Plague.* (Amhearst, NY: Prometheus Books), 33, 35, 88.

Spotlight, The. 1982. January 18. [Defunct newsletter.]

Squires, S. 1989. The Other Side of Thalidomide. *Washington Post,* June 20, Z09.

Stanton, D. 2016. Sanofi Abandoning Auvi-Q after Dosage Problems Led to Total Recall. *In-PharmaTechnologist,* Feb. 23. http://www.in-pharmatechnologist .com/Processing/Sanofi-abandoning-Auvi-Q-after-dosage-problems-led-to -total-recall, acc. Sep. 18, 2017.

Steering Committee of the Physicians' Health Study Research Group. 1989. Final Report on the Aspirin Component of the Ongoing Physicians' Health Study. *New England Journal of Medicine,* July 20;321(3): 129–35.

Stene, LC, J Ulriksen, P Magnus, et al. 2000. Use of Cod Liver Oil During Pregnancy Associated with Lower Risk of Type I Diabetes in the Offspring. *Diabetologia,* Sep.;43(9): 1093–98.

Stein, R. 2007. FDA Delay in Cancer Therapy Is Attacked. *Washington Post,* July 6.

Steinreich, D. 2005. Playing God at the FDA. June 2. https://mises.org/library /playing-god-fda, acc. Nov. 5, 2017.

StreetInsider.com. 2016. NephroGenex (NRX) to Pause Clinical Program of Product Candidate Oral Pyridorin for Treatment of Diabetic Nephropathy. Feb. 24. http://www.streetinsider.com/Corporate+News/NephroGenex +(NRX)+to+Pause+Clinical+Program+of+Product+Candidate+Oral +Pyridorin+for+Treatment+of+Diabetic+Nephropathy/11355289.html, acc. Jan. 29, 2017.

Szabo, L. 2014. FDA Gives Controversial Doc Green Light to Restart Work. *USA Today*, June 25. http://www.usatoday.com/story/news/nation/2014/06/25/burzynski-trial-reopens/11353085/, acc. Mar. 6, 2016.

Tabarrok, AT. 2000. Accessing the FDA via the Anomaly of Off-Label Drug Prescribing. *The Independent Review*, Summer 5(1): 25–53, note 19.

Telser, LG. 1975. The Supply Response to Shifting Demand in the Ethical Pharmaceutical Industry. In *Drug Development and Marketing*, ed. RB Helms. (Washington, DC: American Enterprise Institute for Health Policy Research), 207–23, esp. 223.

Temin, P. 1980. *Taking Your Medicine: Drug Regulation in the United States*. (Cambridge, MA: Harvard University Press), 44, 122, 128, 133–37.

Texas Medical Board vs. Dr. Stanislaw Burzynski, MD, PhD. n.d. Transcript. http://www.burzynskimovie.com/typography/chapter-6-of-10-sourced-transcript/#.WGqK9BsrJEY, acc. Jan. 2, 2017.

Texas Medical Board v. Stanislaw Burzynski Soah Docket No. 503-14-1342.MD, Proposal for Decision, Oct. 12, 2016. http://www.burzynskimovie.com/wpcontent/uploads/2016/10/Proposal_for_Decision_DrB_2016.pdf, acc. Jan. 2, 2017.

Texas State Office of Administrative Hearings. 2015. Second Amended Complaint, Stanislaw Burzynski v. Texas Medical Board SOAH Docket No. 503-14-1342, License No. n-9377. Sep. 24, 2015.

Thomas, GN, OB Hartaigh, JA Bosch, et al. 2012. Vitamin D Levels Predict All-Cause and Cardiovascular Disease Mortality in Subjects with the Metabolic Syndrome: The Ludwigshafen Risk and Hossein-Nezhad and Holick Mayo Health (LURIC) Study. *Diabetes Care*, May;35(5): 1158–64.

Thomas, LG. 1990. Regulation and Firm Size: FDA Impacts on Innovation. *Rand Journal of Economics*, 21(4): 497–517, esp. 514, Appendix.

Throckmorton, DC. 2014. Non-Clinical Cardiovascular Safety Testing: Moving Forward. Oct. 22, 6. http://www.fda.gov/downloads/aboutfda/centersoffices/officeofmedicalproductsandtobacco/cder/ucm420834.pdf, acc. May 15, 2016.

Thun, MJ, EJ Jacobs, & C Patrono. 2012. The Role of Aspirin in Cancer Prevention. *Nature Reviews Clinical Oncology*, Apr.3;9(5): 259–67.

Topol, EJ. 2004. Failing the Public Health—Rofecoxib, Merck, and the FDA. *New England Journal of Medicine*, Oct. 21;351(17): 1707–09.

Trowbridge, RL, & S Walker. 2007. The FDA's Deadly Track Record. *Wall Street Journal*, Aug. 14, A17.

Urology Times. 2009. Immunotherapy Significantly Prolongs Survival in Men with Advanced Prostate Ca. Apr. 29. http://urologytimes.modernmedicine.com

/urology-times/news/clinical/urology/immunotherapy-significantly
-prolongs-survival-men-advanced-prost, acc. Jan. 22, 2018.

US Census Bureau. 1994. Table No. 138: Life Years Lost and Mortality Costs, by Age, Sex, and Cause: 1991. In *Statistical Abstract of the United States*. (Washington, DC: US Government Printing Office), 102.

———. 2004. Table No. 112. *Statistical Abstract of the United States*. (Washington, DC: US Government Printing Office).

———. 2012a. Table 117. *Statistical Abstract of the United States*. (Washington, DC: US Government Printing Office), 103. https://www2.census.gov/library /publications/2011/compendia/statab/131ed/2012-statab.pdf, acc. Sep. 10, 2017.

———. 2012b. Table No. 159. *Statistical Abstract of the United States*. (Washington, DC: US Government Printing Office), 113. http://www2.census.gov/library /publications/2011/compendia/statab/131ed/tables/health.pdf, acc. June 11, 2016.

US Code. 1962. S.1552, Drug Amendments of 1962: Public Law 87-78, Oct. 10. http://uscode.house.gov/statutes/pl/87/781.pdf, acc. Oct. 23, 2017.

US Congress. 2017a. S.204—Trickett Wendler, Frank Mongiello, Jordan McLinn, and Matthew Bellina. Right to Try Act of 2017. https://www.congress.gov /bill/115th-congress/senate-bill/204, acc. Nov. 12, 2017.

———. 2017b. HR 2810—National Defense Authorization Act for Fiscal Year 2018. https://www.congress.gov/bill/115th-congress/house-bill/2810/text?q =%7B%22search%22%3A%5B%22H.r.+2810+section+732%22%5D %7D&r=2, acc. Nov. 11, 2017.

———. 2017c. HR 2117—Health Freedom Protection Act. https://www.congress .gov/bill/110th-congress/house-bill/2117/text, acc. Nov. 11, 2017.

US Court of Appeals, DC Circuit. 1991. 930 F.2d 72, 289 U.S.App.D.C. 187, Barr Laboratories Inc., Petitioners. No. 90-1402. http://openjurist.org/930/f2d/72 /in-re-barr-laboratories-incs, acc. Feb. 9, 2016.

———. 2004. Julian Whitaker, et al., Appellants, V. Tommy G. Thompson, Secretary, US Department of Health and Human Services, et al., Appellees. Jan. 9. http://openjurist.org/353/f3d/947, acc. Jan. 12, 2014.

———. 2006. Abigail Alliance for Better Access to Developmental Drugs and Washington Legal Foundation, Appellants, v. Andrew C. Von Eschenbach, M.D., in His Official Capacity as Acting Commissioner, Food and Drug Administration, and Michael O. Leavitt, in His Official Capacity as Secretary, US Dept. of Health and Human Services, Appellees, No. 04-5350. US Court of Appeals, District of Columbia Circuit. May 2. http://caselaw.findlaw.com /us-dc-circuit/1324774.html, acc. Aug. 29, 2017.

———. 2007. 495 F.3d 695. Abigail Alliance for Better Access to Developmental Drugs and Washington Legal Foundation, Appellants v. Andrew Von Eschenbach, in His Official Capacity as Commissioner, Food and Drug Administration and Michael O. Leavitt, in His Official Capacity as Secretary, US Dept. of Health and Human Services, Appellees. No. 04-5350. US Court of Appeals, District of Columbia Circuit, Aug. 7. https://scholar.google. com/scholar_case?case=8342520538153713995&q=Abigail+Alliance+for +Better+Access+to+Developmental+Drugs+v.+von+Eschenbach&hl =en&as_sdt=6,44&as_vis=1, acc. Oct. 28, 2017.

———. 2014. United States of America, Appellee v. Regenerative Sciences, LLC, a Corporation, et al., Appellants. 2014. US Court of Appeals for the District of Columbia Circuit, Feb. 4. https://www.cadc.uscourts.gov/internet/opinions .nsf/0/947528CDDA0B9A5A85257C7500533DF4/$file/12-5254-1478137 .pdf, acc. Jan. 27, 2015.

US District Court for DC. 1999. Durk Pearson and Sandy Shaw, American Preventive Medical Association and Citizens For Health, Appellants v. Donna E. Shalala, Secretary, US Department of Health and Human Services, et al., Appellees. Jan. 15. http://www.emord.com/Emord%20&%20Associates,%20 Pearson%20v.%20Shalala.pdf, acc. Jan. 12, 2014.

US District Court for Delaware. 1970. 307 F. Supp. 858, US District Court for the District of Delaware, Pharmaceutical Manufacturers Association v. Finch. http://law.justia.com/cases/federal/district-courts/FSupp/307/858/1428433/, acc. July 15, 2017.

US Food and Drug Administration (FDA). n.d.a. Drugs@FDA: FDA Approved Drug Products. https://www.accessdata.fda.gov/Scripts/Cder/Daf/Index.cfm? Event=Overview.process&Applno=021430, acc. July 2, 2016.

———. n.d.b. Is It True FDA Is Approving Fewer New Drugs Lately? https://www .fda.gov/downloads/AboutFDA/Transparency/Basics/UCM247465.pdf, acc. Sep. 10, 2017.

———. Annual Ed. *The Orange Book: Approved Drug Products with Therapeutic Equivalence Evaluations.* (Silver Spring, MD: FDA). http://www.accessdata.fda .gov/scripts/cder/ob/docs/obdetail.cfm?Appl_No=018859&TABLE1=OB _Rx, acc. May 25, 2016.

———. 1991. Antiviral Advisory Committee Meeting. Feb. 13–14. Personal communication.

———. 1996. Food Standards: Amendment of Standards of Identity for Enriched Grain Products to Require Addition of Folic Acid. Final Rule. *Federal Register* 61(44): 8781–97.

———. 1998. FDA "Approvable" Letter to Celegene. July 16. http://www.accessdata .fda.gov/drugsatfda_docs/appletter/1998/20785ltr.pdf, acc. July 2, 2016.

———. 2005a. *CDER 2005 Report to the Nation: Improving Public Health Through Human Drugs.* (Rockville, MD: US Food and Drug Administration), 42, 43.

———. 2005b. Warning Letter to Cherry Republic, Oct. 17. http://www.fda.gov /iceci/enforcementactions/warningletters/2005/ucm075633.htm, acc. on Nov. 23, 2013.

———. 2009. Warning Letter to General Mills, May 5. http://www.fda.gov/iceci /enforcementactions/warningletters/2009/ucm162943.htm, acc. Nov. 23, 2013.

———. 2010a. Approval Letter, Apr. 29. Provenge. http://www.fda.gov/biologics- bloodvaccines/cellulargenetherapyproducts/approvedproducts/ucm210215 .htm, acc. Dec 15, 2015.

———. 2010b. Warning Letter to Diamond Foods. Feb. 22. http://www.fda.gov /ICECI/EnforcementActions/WarningLetters/ucm202825.htm, acc. Nov. 23, 2013.

———. 2011. Comments of the Alliance for Natural Health USA. In *re Draft Guidance for Industry; Dietary Supplements: New Dietary Ingredients Notifi- cations and Related Issues; Availability; Extension of Comment Period* (76 Fed. Reg. 9111), FDA Docket No. 2011-D-0376-1603, at 12 (Dec. 2, 2011).

———. 2014. Human Cells, Tissues, and Cellular and Tissue-Based Products (HCT/ Ps) from Adipose Tissue: Regulatory Considerations, Draft Guidance, Dec. http://www.fda.gov/BiologicsBloodVaccines/GuidanceComplianceRegulatory Information/Guidances/Tissue/ucm427795.htm, acc. Oct. 2, 2016.

———. 2016. FDA News Release: FDA Grants Accelerated Approval to First Drug for Duchenne Muscular Dystrophy. Sep. 19, 2016. http://www.fda.gov /newsevents/newsroom/pressannouncements/ucm521263.htm, acc. Jan. 1, 2017.

———. 2017a. Prescription Drug User Fee Act (PDUFA). https://www.fda.gov/ forindustry/userfees/prescriptiondruguserfee/default.htm, acc. Oct. 30, 2017.

———. 2017b. FY 2016 PDUFA Financial Report. pp. 9, 16. https://www.fda.gov /downloads/AboutFDA/ReportsManualsForms/Reports/UserFeeReports /FinancialReports/PDUFA/UCM550408.pdf, acc. Oct. 31, 2017.

———. 2018. Expanded Access (Compassionate Use). https://www.fda.gov /NewsEvents/PublicHealthFocus/ExpandedAccessCompassionateUse /default.htm, acc. Jan. 22, 2018.

US Patent. 1962. Patent #3,069,322. Issued Dec. 18, 1962.

———. 2008. Compositions and Methods for the Treatment of Radiation Burns and Other Traumatic Skin Conditions. US Patent #7, 390,507. Issued June 24, 2008.

US Supreme Court. 1911. SCT.248, 221 US 488, 55 L. Ed. 823, 31 S. Ct. 627, Supreme Court of the United States. United States v. Johnson, May 29, 1911. http://drug library.org/schaffer/legal/l1910/Usvjohnson.htm, acc. July 15, 2017.

Vandvik, PO, DD Gutterman, P Alonso-Coello, et al. 2012. Primary and Secondary Prevention of Cardiovascular Disease Antithrombotic Therapy and Prevention of Thrombosis, 9th ed. American College of Chest Physicians Evidence-Based Clinical Practice Guidelines. *Chest*;141(2) (Suppl): e637S–e668S.

Vavra, JJ. 1967. Development of Resistance to Novobiocin, Tetracycline, and a Novobiocin-Tetracycline Combination in Staphylococcus Aureus Populations. *Journal of Bacteriology*, Mar.;93(3): 801–05.

Vermorken, JB, R Mesia, F Rivera, et al. 2008. Platinum-based Chemotherapy Plus Cetuximab in Head and Neck Cancer. *New England Journal of Medicine*, Sep. 11;359(11): 1116–27.

Vernon, JA, JH Golec, & JA DiMasi. 2010. Drug Development Costs When Financial Risk Is Measured Using the Fama-French Three-Factor Model. *Health Economics*, 19(8): 1002–05.

Viereck, C., & P Boudes. 2011. An Analysis of the Impact of FDA's Guidelines for Addressing Cardiovascular Risk of Drugs for Type 2 Diabetes on Clinical Development. *Contemporary Clinical Trials*, May;32 (3): 324–32.

Wall Street Journal. 1988. FDA Now Formally Allows Personal-Use Drug Imports. July 25, p. 39.

Wang, C. 2013. Role of Vitamin D in Cardiometabolic Diseases. *Journal of Diabetes Research*, 243934. Epub, Feb. 25.

Wardell, WM. 1978. The Rate of Development of New Drugs in the United States. *Clinical Pharmacology and Therapeutics*, Aug;24(2): 133–45.

———. 1979. Rx: More Regulation or Better Therapies? *Regulation*, 1979 Sept/ Oct.;3(5): 25–33, esp. 30.

———. 1983. Hearings on Pharmaceutical Patent Life and Innovation. Submitted to the Subcommittee on Investigations and Oversight of the Committee on Science and Technology, US House of Representatives, Feb. 4, 1982. (Washington, DC: US Government Printing Office).

Wardell, WM, & L Lasagna. 1975. *Regulation and Drug Development*. (Washington, DC: American Enterprise Institute for Public Policy Research), 13, 15–16, 20, 22, 50–77.

Wardell, WM, M May, & G Trimble. 1982. New Drug Development by the United States Pharmaceutical Firms with Analyses of Trends in the Acquisition and Origin of Drug Candidates, 1963–1979. *Clinical Pharmacology and Therapeutics*, Oct.;32(4).

Wasseman, E. 2016. Merck Reaches $830M Settlement in Long-Running Vioxx Litigation. Jan 15. http://www.fiercepharma.com/regulatory/merck-reaches-830m-settlement-long-running-vioxx-litigation, acc. Feb. 3, 2017.

Watson, JD. 1965. *Molecular Biology of the Gene*. (New York: W. A. Benjamin). https://www.abebooks.co.uk/servlet/BookDetailsPL?bi=22053432180&searchurl=tn%3Dmolecular%2Bbiology%2Bof%2Bthe%2Bgene%26sortby%3D17%26an%3Dwatson%2Bjames%26fe%3Don&cm_sp=snippet-_-srp1-_-title2.

Wegner, HC. 2014. *Patent Law in Biotechnology, Chemicals, and Pharmaceuticals*. (Basingstoke, United Kingdom: Palgrave Macmillan): 301.

Weiss, J. 2008. *Business Ethics: A Stakeholder and Issues Management Approach*. 5th ed. (Boston: Cengage Learning), 199.

Wiggins, SN. 1981. Product Quality Regulation and New Drug Introductions: Some New Evidence from the 1970s. *Review of Economics and Statistics*;63(4): 615–19.

Wikipedia. n.d.a. United States Military Casualties of War. https://en.wikipedia.org/wiki/United_States_military_casualties_of_war, acc. Oct. 30, 2017.

———. n.d.b. List of Withdrawn Drugs. http://en.wikipedia.org/wiki/List_of_withdrawn_drugs, acc. Oct. 25, 2013.

Wilkerson Group. 1996. Forces Reshaping the Performance and Contribution of the US Medical Device Industry. Prepared for the Health Industry Manufacturers Association. Cited in RD Tollison, "Institutional Alternatives for the Regulation of Drugs and Medical Devices." In *Advancing Medical Innovation: Health, Safety, and the Role of Government in the 21st Century*, eds. RA Epstein, TM Lenard, HI Miller, et al. (Washington, DC: Progress and Freedom Foundation).

Williams, L. 1992. F.D.A. Steps Up Effort to Control Vitamin Claims. *New York Times*, Aug. 9. http://www.nytimes.com/1992/08/09/us/fda-steps-up-effort-to-control-vitamin-claims.html?pagewanted=all, acc. Nov. 2, 2017.

Willingham, E. 2016. Why Did Mylan Hike Epipen Prices 400%? Because They Could. *Forbes.* Aug. 21. https://www.forbes.com/sites/emilywillingham /2016/08/21/why-did-mylan-hike-epipen-prices-400-because-they-could /#384e9072280c, acc. Sep. 18, 2017.

Wilson, S. 1942. *Food and Drug Regulation.* (Washington, DC: American Council on Public Affairs), 22–23, 27.

Wright, J. 1992. *FDA vs. the People of the United States: Five Years of Assault on "Self-Care."* (Tacoma, WA: Jonathan Wright Legal Defense Fund).

Wright, JV, & L Lenard. 2009. Stay Young and Sexy with Bio-Identical Hormone Replacement: The Science Explained Natural Hormone Replacement for Women over 45. (Walnut, CA: Smart Publications).

Yang, W, TM Dall, P Halder, et al. 2013. Economic Costs of Diabetes in the US in 2012. *Diabetes Care,* Apr.;36(4): 1033–46.

Yarchoan, R, RW Klecker, KJ Weinhold, et al. 1986. Administration of 3'-Azi-do-3'Deoxythymidine, An Inhibitor of HTLV-III/LAV Replication, to Patients with AIDS or AIDS-related Complex. *Lancet,* Mar. 15;1(8481): 575–80.

Yarema, MC, DW Johnson, RJ Berlin, et al. 2009. Comparison of the 20-hour Intravenous and 72-hour Oral Acetylcysteine Protocols for the Treatment of Acute Acetaminophen Poisoning. *Annals of Emergency Medicine,* Oct.;54(4): 606–14.

Young, SD. 1987. *The Rule of Experts.* (Washington, DC: Cato Institute), 16.

Xu, J, SL Murphy, KD Kochanek, et al. 2016. Deaths: Final Data for 2011. *National Vital Statistics Report*;64(2). http://origin.glb.cdc.gov/nchs/data/nvsr/nvsr64 /nvsr64_02.pdf, acc. June 4, 2016.

Zandonella, C. 2013. Drug-Resistant MRSA Bacteria: Here to Stay in Both Hospital and Community. *Science Daily,* Mar. 15. http://www.sciencedaily.com /releases/2013/03/130315202724.htm, acc. Mar. 30, 2017.

Zhang, G, N Shirai, T Higuchi, et al. 2007. Effect of Erabu Sea Snake (Laticauda semifasciata) Lipids on the Swimming Endurance of Aged Mice. *Journal of Nutritional Science and Vitaminology* (Tokyo), Dec.;53(6): 476–81.

Zheng, Y, J Zhu, M Zhou, et al. 2013. Meta-Analysis of Long-Term Vitamin D Supplementation on Overall Mortality. *PLOS ONE,* 8(12): e82109.

Zittermann, A, SS Schleithoff, & R Koerfer. 2005. Putting Cardiovascular Disease and Vitamin D Insufficiency into Perspective. *British Journal of Nutrition,* Oct.;94(4): 483–92.

Zlatohlavek, L, M Vrablik, B Grauova, et al. 2012. The Effect of Coenzyme Q10 in Statin Myopathy. *Neuro Endocrinology Letters,* 33 Suppl 2: 98–101.

Index

A

Abbreviated New Drug Application (ANDA), 97

AbbVie, 93–95

Abigail Alliance, 36, 45, 218–19, 226–27

abortion, 196

access to drugs
for cancer, 36–37, 207–8, 210, 219
lack of, deaths from, 43–47
"Right to Try" legislation, 219
terminally ill patients, 19–21, 35–37, 200, 219

acetaminophen, 187–88

acquired immune deficiency syndrome drugs. *See* AIDS drugs

acyclovir, 82

Adamis, 99

Adrenaclick, 100

advertising
about prevention, 171
cautions included in, 26, 91
compounded products, 93

FDA approval of, 55, 90–91
medical information in, 164–65
natural products, 162, 181–85
scenario without Amendments, 219–20

aerosolized pentamidine, 70–71

age-related macular degeneration (AMD), 191

AHFS. *See* American Hospital Formulary Service (AHFS)

AIDS drugs. *See also specific drugs*
approvals of, 61–72
black market for, 32–34, 64, 71, 208, 210, 218
combination therapy for, 13
success of, 124

Aiken, James W., 76

allergies, 99–100

alprostadil, 196

ALS. *See* amyotrophic lateral sclerosis (ALS)

AMA. *See* American Medical Association (AMA)

Amarin, 189

AMD. *See* age-related macular degeneration (AMD)

American Heart Association, 78

American Hospital Formulary Service (AHFS), 225

American Medical Association (AMA), 112, 139, 224–25

"American thalidomide," 3, 163–65, 204, 230

amyotrophic lateral sclerosis (ALS), 129–30, 218–19

ANDA. *See* Abbreviated New Drug Application (ANDA)

Androgel®, 93–95

andropause, 93–95

angina, 81

angiogenesis, 195

animal testing

    alternatives to, 96

    anti-inflammatory agents, 154–55

    aspirin, 76

    FDA requirements for, 28, 48–51

    limits of, 25–26

    nutrition and, 157–58

    pentamidine, 70

    thalidomide, 25

anthrax, 104

anti-AIDS drugs, 33, 124

antibiotics

    bacterial resistance to, 12–14, 102–3

    combinations of, 12–15, 127, 198

    discovery of, 102

    new development of, 103–4

    patents for, 104

    side effects of, 143–44

anti-cancer drugs. *See also specific drugs*

    access to, 36–37, 207–8, 210, 219

    number of, 40–41

anti-hypertensive agents, 40, 52–53, 81, 171

anti-inflammatory drugs, 54, 76, 148–49. *See also specific drugs*

anti-neoplastons, 133–36

anti-obesity drugs, 54

anti-oxidants, 161–62, 180, 188

anti-toxins, 132

anti-viral drugs, 61–72. *See also* AIDS drugs; *specific drugs*

approvals

    generic drugs, 97

    as guarantees, 26, 28–31, 198, 213–14

    health care costs and, 125

    lives saved by, 43–44, 121

    of orphan drugs. *See* Orphan Drug Act

    political influences on, 61–72, 148–54

    and the race to market, 16, 35–36, 84

    review time, 74, 82

    revocation of FDA's authority for, 216–20

    risk-to-benefit assessment, 27

    scenario without, 232–39

    US-based studies requirement, 41, 52, 62

Arizona, 82

arthritis, 148

aspirin, 75–82, 111, 122, 149, 156, 205

assays, 49–50, 62

auto-immune diseases, 167

automation, 96
Auvi-Q, 99–100
AZT (azidothymidine), 61–64

B
Bailey, Joanna Shepherd, 194
balding, 171–72
Bandow, Doug, 126
Barre-National, 17
Barr Laboratories, 17
Bayer, 104, 158
Bayh-Dole Act, 105–6
benzoquinone, 132
beta-blockers, 39–40
bioequivalence studies, 97
bio-identical HRT, 177
Biostratum Inc., 192
birth defects
    folic acid, 3, 163–65, 180, 204, 230
    thalidomide, 1, 3, 9–10, 25, 144–45, 212
black market
    AIDS drugs, 32–34, 64, 71, 208, 210, 218
blood pressure medicine, 40, 52–53, 81, 171
blood tests for HIV, 71–72
blue babies, 196
Bonnville, Dimitri, 127
brand-name drugs. *See also specific drugs*
    customer loyalty to, 8, 230
    versus generic drugs, 7–8
    prices for, 88–89
breast cancer, 172–74
breast reconstruction, 130–31
bribery, 17, 199

Brimelow, Peter, 18
Britain. *See* United Kingdom
burn cream, 172–74
Burroughs, Abigail, 36
Burroughs, Frank, 36, 45
Burroughs-Wellcome, 63, 69
Burzynski, Stanislaw, 133–36, 236
Bush, George H. W., 68
Buyers Clubs, 32–34, 64

C
calcium, 168, 169
cancer patients. *See also specific type of cancer*
    access to drugs, 36–37, 207–8, 210, 219
    death rates, 44–45
    new therapies for, 41–42, 132–37, 203, 236
    number of drugs for, 40–41
capitalized costs, 88–89, 92–93
cardiovascular disease
    aspirin for, 75–79, 111, 122, 205
    drug-induced, 148–56
    heart attacks. *See* heart attacks
    hypercholesterolemia, 183, 186–87
    hypertension, 40, 52–53, 81, 171
    new drugs for, 39–40, 44, 110–11
    off-label use for, 80–81, 205
    vitamin D and, 168–69
CD4$^+$ assays, 62, 65
CDC. *See* Centers for Disease Control and Prevention (CDC)
Celebrex, 151, 153
cellular therapy, 117–20
Centeno, Christopher, 128–29

Centers for Disease Control and Prevention (CDC), 70, 163–64
cerebrovascular disease, 44, 75, 79, 148
certification, 222–28
certifying agencies, 221
Cheerios, 183
Chemie Grüenthal, 9
cherries, 182–83
chloramphenicol, 143–44
cholesterol, 183, 186–87
Christopher, William, 83
Ciba Geigy, 20
cimetidine, 124
Cipro, 104
CMV. *See* cytomegalovirus retinitis (CMV) virus
cod liver oil, 166, 189–91, 231
coenzyme Q10, 177, 186–87
colorectal cancer, 69, 81, 180
combination products
    antibiotics, 12–15, 127, 198
    FDA resistance to, 155
    natural products and drugs, 186–88
    scenario without Amendments, 209, 237
commercial speech, 29, 55, 171
"compassionate use," 21, 35–37
compounding pharmacies, 93–95
computers, 96
Congress
    antibiotic development incentives, 104
    Burzynski case, 134
    FDA censure by, 28–31, 213–14
Congressional Budget Office, 90
Constitution, First Amendment, 29, 55, 82, 171, 180

consumers
    brand-name loyalty, 8, 230
    drug prices for. *See* prices
    informed decisions by, 217–18, 221, 226, 237
    reviews by, 223–28, 230
consumer groups, 226–27. *See also specific group*
ConsumerLab.com, 227
Consumer Reports, 227
Consumers' Research, 225
Cooper, Ellen, 67
Corbitt, Earl, 134
CorePharma, 98
corruption, 17–18, 57, 197–99, 202
Cotto, Josia, 135
court rulings
    cancer treatments, 134–36
    expanded access, 36–37
    FDA power, 15, 28, 198, 216–17
    FDA refusal to obey, 179–81, 198, 217
    health claims, 23–24, 181, 217
    stem cell research, 129
COX inhibitors, 149, 153, 154
Cox, David, 67
Crout, Richard, 133
Cutter vaccine, 143–45
cytomegalovirus retinitis (CMV) virus, 68–69
cytoprotection, 155

D
Dallas Buyers Club (movie), 33
daraprim, 98–99
DCB. *See* device certifying body (DCB)
ddC, 33–34

deaths
  from Amendments, 146–48, 200–202
  from cancer, 44–45
  from development delays, 45–46, 200–201
  drug-induced, 147–48, 202, 237
  heart attack, 44
  infection, 101–2
  from lack of access to drugs, 43–47
  from loss of innovation, 121–23, 201
  from paradigm shift, 123
Defense Department, 219–20
Delaney, Martin, 64, 66
Delpassand, Ebrahim, 219
Dendron Pharmaceuticals, 117–20
dermatomyo-fibromas, 174
development process
  cost of, 39, 56, 73–74, 84–87
    impact on prices, 50, 54, 88–91, 201, 235–36
    recovery of, 105, 108–9, 113–14, 202
    without Amendments, 92–96
  delays in, 39–41
    deaths from, 45–46, 200–201
  FDA power over, 28
  impact on research, 79, 105–6, 203
  scenario without FDA approval, 232–39
  time required for, 16, 29–31, 38–39, 48–55, 84–87
  withdrawals from, 55, 86, 91, 108–9, 113–14, 121–22, 140–42
device certifying body (DCB), 224
DHA. See docosahexaenoic acid (DHA)

diabetes, 31, 54, 167–68, 193
Diamond Foods, 184–85
Diet. See health behavior; nutrition
Dietary Supplement Health and Education Act of 1994 (DSHEA), 192–94, 204
diethylene glycol, 225
docosahexaenoic acid (DHA), 191
doctors. See physicians
Donsabch, Kurt, 175
drugs. See also specific drugs
  access to. See access to drugs
  advertising of. See advertising
  brand name. See brand-name drugs
  certification of, 222–28
  deaths caused by, 147–48, 202, 237
  effectiveness of. See effectiveness
  generic. See generic drugs
  information about. See information
  interactions between, 147–48, 202, 237
  manufacturing of. See manufacturing process
  natural products classified as, 181–85, 204–5, 217, 219–20
  natural products combined with, 186–88
  natural products replaced by, 104, 161–62, 170
  new. See new chemical entities
  price of. See prices
  safety of. See safety
drug companies. See pharmaceutical industry; specific companies
Drug Efficacy Study (National Academy of Sciences), 11–15, 23, 138–39

Drug Information Clinical Database, 225

DSHEA. *See* Dietary Supplement Health and Education Act of 1994 (DSHEA)

Duchenne's disease, 232–35

ductus arteriosus, 196

E

effectiveness

  approvals as guarantee of, 26, 28–31, 198, 213–14

  definition of, 23–27

  effect of Amendments on, 138–40

  evaluation of, 11–15, 23, 138–40

  individual differences in, 139–40, 196, 211, 236–37

  natural product, 162, 180

  standards for, 14, 51–54, 70

eicosanoids. *See* prostaglandins

eicosapentaenoic acid (EPA), 191

electrical appliances, 223, 226

Elias, Thomas D., 135

Elixir Sulfanilamide, 224–25

Emord, Jonathan, 80, 193

Emory University, 129

EPA. *See* eicosapentaenoic acid (EPA)

epinephrine, 99–100

Epi-Pen, 99–100

Erbitux, 36

erectile dysfunction, 196

eteplirsen, 233–35

ethics

  corruption, 17–18, 57, 197–99, 202

  placebo effect, 63, 69, 77, 233

  price gouging, 97–100, 203

  user fees, 150–52, 180, 202–4, 236

Europe. *See also specific countries*

  approval process in, 224

  mifamurtide in, 20

  new drugs in, 41–42, 116, 142

  thalidomide tragedy in, 1, 3, 9–10, 25, 145, 212

Exondys, 235

expanded access programs, 21, 35–37

F

Faloon, Bill, 178

fatty acid esters, 189–91

FDA. *See* Food and Drug Administration (FDA)

Federal Trade Commission, 219–20

F. Hoffmann-La Roche AG, 158

fiber, dietary, 180

financial analysis, 59–60, 202, 229–30

"first-in-class" drug candidates, 111

first-to-market drugs, 16, 35–36, 84

fish oil, 189–91, 204, 231

Florida, 177–78

flu, 101–2

folic acid, 3, 163–65, 180–81, 204, 230

folk medicine, 231. *See also* natural products

Food and Drug Act 1938, amendments to. *See* Kefauver-Harris Amendments

Food and Drug Administration (FDA)

  bias against physicians developing drugs, 132–33, 176–77

  as certifying agency, 226

  corruption within, 17–18, 57, 197–99, 202

  court orders, refusal to obey, 179–81, 198, 217

dismantling of, 215
drug approvals. *See* approvals
effectiveness evaluation. *See* effectiveness
political influences, 61–72, 148–54
powers of, 2, 16–22, 28, 198, 216–17
raids by, 175–78
reform of, 236
retaliation against drug companies, 29, 65, 219, 238
as scapegoat, 28–31, 198, 213–14
user fees, 30, 140–41, 150–52, 180, 202–4, 236
warning letters to food producers, 182–85
foods. *See also* natural products
as drugs, 182–85, 205, 217, 219–20
Franklin, Benjamin, 157
Frazier, Kenneth, 59
freedom, 211, 220, 226, 237
free speech, 55, 82, 171, 180, 218
Freund, John, 54

G
Gallo, Robert C., 64
ganciclovir, 68–69
Garabedian, Chris, 233–35
gastric ulcers, 124, 149, 154–55
gastrointestinal infections, 101–2
General Federation of Women's Clubs, 225
generic drugs. *See also specific drugs*
corruption scandal, 17
development costs, 94, 97
history of, 7–8
patents and, 73–74, 97
prices of, 97–100

Gieringer, Dale, 142, 143, 156
Ginn, Lesli G., 136
Glasky, Alvin J., 64–65
Glaxo, 189
GlaxoSmithKline, 98
glutathione, 188
glyoxilide, 132
GMPs. *See* Good Manufacturing Practices (GMPs)
Golden Age of Health
concept of, 3–4
creation of, 215–21, 238–39
effect of Amendments on, 199, 206, 214
Goldwater Institute, 219
Good Housekeeping, 227
Good Manufacturing Practices (GMPs), 55, 57–59, 194, 198
Graham, David, 150–51, 153
Grant, William B., 169, 170
Grüenthal GmbH, 9

H
Harada, Ted, 129
health behavior, 44–45, 79, 158, 237–38
health care costs, 124–26
health claims
as basis for drug classification, 171, 181–85, 217–18
effectiveness and, 162
scenario without Amendments, 209, 220–21
health food stores, FDA raids of, 175–78
Health Freedom Protection Act (HR 2117), 220–21
health insurance, 236

heart attacks. *See also* cardiovascular
disease
death rates from, 44
drug-induced, 148, 153
prevention of, 44, 76–78, 168–69, 189
stem cell therapy, 127–28
hemophilia, 71
Henderson, David R., 21, 226
herbal remedies, 231. *See also* natural products
high blood pressure, 40, 52–53, 81, 171
high cholesterol, 183, 186–87
HIV, 13, 62.
blood tests for, 71–72
Hoffman, Freddie Ann, 134
Hoffmann-LaRoche, 34
Holick, Michael F., 167
hormone replacement therapy (HRT), 177
Hoxey, Harry, 132
Hoxey Herbal Therapy, 132
HRT. *See* hormone replacement therapy (HRT)
human immunodeficiency virus. *See* HIV
human studies
ethical issues with, 63, 69, 77, 233
FDA power over, 28
limits of, 25–26
number of people in, 53
Phase 1 trials, 51
Phase 2 trials, 51
Phase 3 trials, 51–54, 193
Phase 4 trials, 55, 87
statistical significance, 52–54, 108, 118
US-based requirement, 41, 52, 62

work burden, 54
Humulin, 30–31
hypercholesterolemia, 183, 186–87
hypertension, 40, 52–53, 81, 171

I
ibuprofen, 149, 155, 156
ICN Pharmaceuticals, 66–68
IDM Pharma, 20
immune stimulants, 61–72, 81, 195. *See also* AIDS drugs; *specific drugs*
Impax, 98
imported drugs, 32–34, 64–66, 200, 208
indications
new, 75–79, 82, 147
off-label use, 80–83, 205
indomethacin, 154
INDs. *See* investigational new drugs (INDs)
infection
deaths caused by, 101–2
drugs for. *See* antibiotics
natural products for, 104
information
about natural products, 180, 190, 204–5, 218
about new indications, 75–82
about nutrition, 166–70
about prevention, 44–45, 171–74
in advertising, 26, 91, 164–65
package inserts, 90–91, 150
restrictions on, 29, 81–82, 171–74
sources of, 225–28
informed decisions, 217–18, 221, 226, 237
innovation
barriers to, 117–20

importance of, 101–4
industry decisions about, 107–9
loss of, 110–14
deaths from, 121–23, 201
by physicians
cancer treatments, 132–37, 203, 236
stem cell research, 127–31, 203
scenario without Amendments,
209–11, 232–39
in United Kingdom, 115–16
university-industry collaboration,
105–6
insulin, 30–31
insurance, 236
Internet, consumer reviews on, 223–28,
230
investigational new drugs (INDs), 35–
37, 192–93
in vitro testing, 48–49, 96
isoprinosine, 32, 64–66
Ivey, Andrew C., 132

J
Japan, 71
Jenner Therapeutics, 20
Jobs, Steve, 41
Jondrow, James, 139

K
Kaiser Permanente, 151
Kaposi's sarcoma, 195
Kefauver, Estes, 7–8
Kefauver-Harris Amendments
changes introduced by, 2, 7–10
FDA powers, 2, 16–22, 28, 198,
216–17. See also Food
and Drug Administration

safety provisions. See safety
cost-benefit analysis, 138–56
deaths caused by, 146–48,
200–202
effectiveness, 138–40
international comparison,
141–42
lives saved, 143–46
prevention versus treatment,
189–91, 200–206
of regulations, 205–6, 212–13
safety, 140–42, 146–48, 201
Vioxx disaster, 148–56, 209,
229–30
enactment of, 1–2, 10
problems caused by, 2–4, 56–60
loss of innovation. See innovation
prevention versus treatment.
See paradigm shift
reasons for, 211–13
remedies for, 215–21
whistleblowers, 5–6, 17, 21
repeal of, 216, 219
scenario without, 209–11, 232–39
thalidomide tragedy as trigger for,
9–10, 145
Kelsey, Frances, 9–10
Kent, Saul, 178
kidney disease, 193
Koch, William Frederick, 132
Krebiozen, 132
KV Pharmaceutical, 93–95

L
labeling, 55, 218
labor induction, 196

Lake, Simeon, 135
LaMattina, John L., 59
Lasagna, Louis, 18, 61
lazeroids, 161–62
LD50 testing, 49
LEF. *See* Life Extension Foundation (LEF)
legal responsibility, 213–15
legislation
    Bayh-Dole Act, 105–6
    Dietary Supplement Health and Education Act, 192–94, 204
    Food and Drug Act amendments. *See* Kefauver-Harris Amendments
    National Defense Authorization Act, 219–20
    Nutrition Labeling and Education Act, 180
    Prescription Drug User Fee Act, 30, 140–41, 150–52, 180, 202–4, 236
    "Right to Try" legislation, 219
    Waxman Hatch Patent Restoration Act, 74, 236
leprosy, 195
levamisole, 81
Ley, Herbert, 5
Lichtenberg, Frank, 43–44, 121
life expectancy, 43–44, 121, 126
Life Extension Foundation (LEF), 177–78, 227–28
lifestyle, impact of 44–45, 79, 158, 237–38
Lincoln, Robert E., 132
liver disease, 107–9, 111, 113, 122, 188
Long, Edward V., 175, 179
Lou Gehrig's disease, 129–30, 218–19

Lovaza, 190
Lyphomed, 70

M
Makena®, 94
male menopause, 93–95
Mansell, Peter, 67
manufacturing versus compounding, 95
    of natural products, 194
    regulation of, 55, 57–59, 91, 198
    of vitamins, 158–59
market leaders, 16, 35–36, 84
mass media campaigns, 164
Max Planck Institute, 62
McDonald, Gabrielle, 134
McNary, Austin, 234
McNary, Jenn, 233–35
Mead, Margaret, 238
medical device manufacturers, 224
The Medical Letter on Drugs and Therapeutics, 225
MER-29, 143–44
Merck, 59, 151, 153, 158, 229–30
mergers, 56, 59
methicillin-resistant *Staphylococcus aureus* (MRSA), 102–3
"me-too" drugs, 111
Mexico, 65, 66
Meyers, Paul, 20
mifamurtide, 19–21
Miller, Henry I., 2, 17, 30–31
minoxidil, 171–72
monoclonal antibodies, 41
Moss, Marion, 176
Motrin®, 149
MRSA. *See* methicillin-resistant *Staphylococcus aureus* (MRSA)

multiple myeloma, 195
multiple sclerosis (MS), 167
multivitamins, 158–59
muscle weakness from statins, 187
Mylan, 17, 99–100
Myopathy from statins, 187

N
N-acetyl cysteine, 187–88
naproxen, 153
National Academy of Sciences, Drug
    Efficacy Study, 11–15, 23,
    138–39
National Cancer Institute (NCI), 62–
    63, 68, 110
National Defense Authorization Act for
    Fiscal Year 2018, 219–20
National Institutes of Health (NIH), 62,
    68, 70–71, 77, 119, 145
natural products. *See also specific prod-*
    uct
    certification of, 227
    classified as drugs, 181–85, 204–5,
        217, 219–20
    dietary ingredients regulations,
        192–94, 204
    drugs combined with, 186–88
    FDA raids, 175–76
    FDA refusal to obey court orders
        on, 179–81, 198, 217
    health claims for, 162, 171, 181–85,
        209, 217–18
    information about, 180, 190, 204–
        5, 218
    patents for, 159, 189
    physician knowledge of, 124, 169,
        190, 204–5
    prices of, 211
    replaced by drugs, 104, 161–62,
        170
    scenario without Amendments,
        209–11
    split-label approach to, 218
    vitamins, 158–59
NBEs. *See* new biologically based enti-
    ties (NBEs)
NCEs. *See* new chemical entities (NCEs)
NCI. *See* National Cancer Institute (NCI)
NDAs. *See* New Drug Applications
    (NDAs)
NDI. *See* new dietary ingredient (NDI)
Neiper, Hans, 175
Nelson, David W., 19
NephroGenex Inc., 193
Netherlands, 164
Neuralstem, 130
neural tube defects, 3, 163–65, 180,
    204, 230
neuroendocrine carcinoma, 41–42
new biologically based entities (NBEs),
    41
new chemical entities (NCEs), 30
new dietary ingredient (NDI), 194
New Drug Applications (NDAs), 29–
    31. *See also* approvals
new molecular entities (NMEs), 30
Newport Pharmaceuticals, 64–65
New Zealand, 65
NIH. *See* National Institutes of Health
    (NIH)
NLEA. *See* Nutrition Labeling and Ed-
    ucation Act of 1990 (NLEA)
nutrition, 157–59. *See also natural*
    products; specific nutrients

information about, 166–70

Nutrition Labeling and Education Act of 1990 (NLEA), 180

O

obesity, 54

octreotide, 41–42

Office of Alternative Medicine (OAM), 134

off-label use, 80–83, 205

older drugs

    improvements in, 111

    new indications for, 75–79, 82, 147

    off-label use, 80–83, 205

omega-3 oils

    benefits of, 155–56, 180, 189–91, 231

    indications for, 204

    in walnuts, 184

OmegaRx, 191

O'Neill, William, 127–28

Orabilex, 143

Orphan Drug Act

    overview, 94–96

    pentamidine, 70

    progesterone, 94–95

    scenario without Amendments, 210, 236

osteosarcoma, 19–21

Ostertag, Wofram, 62

outcome studies, 54

ovarian cancer, 208

overseas development, 39–41

overseas importation, 32–34, 64–66, 200, 208

overseas treatment, 42

P

package inserts, 90–91, 150

Panalba, 13–15, 23, 103–4

paradigm shift

    overview, 157–60

    cost-benefit analysis, 189–91, 200–206

    deaths from, 123

    dietary ingredients regulations, 192–94, 204

    FDA raids, 175–78

    information restrictions, 44–45, 171–74

    natural products and. *See* natural products

Pasteur Institute, 62

patents

    antibiotics, 104

    burn cream, 174

    expiration of, 73–74, 97, 108–9, 147

    natural products, 159, 189

    pentamidine, 70

    prostaglandins, 159

    requirement for, 73–74, 160–62, 236

    by universities, 105–6

patients. *See* consumers

Paul, Ron, 219

Pazdur, Richard, 207–8

PCBs. *See* polychlorinated biphenyls (PCBs)

PCP. *See* Pneumocystis pneumonia (PCP)

PDUFA. *See* Prescription Drug User Fee Act (PDUFA)

Pearson, Durk, 218

Peltzman, Sam, 111–12, 139, 142, 145
penicillin, 58
Penrod, Mariss, 234
pentamidine, 69–71
Peptide Receptor Radionuclide Therapy (PRRT), 41–42
Pfizer, 60
PGE1. *See* prostaglandin E$_1$ (PGE1)
PGI$_2$. *See* prostacyclin (PGI$_2$)
pharmaceutical industry. *See also specific companies*
    cartelization of, 57–69, 197–98, 202–3, 210, 213
    drug development by. *See* development process
    expanded access programs, 21, 35–37
    FDA employees hired by, 19
    FDA power over, 2, 16–22, 28, 198, 216–17
    FDA retaliation against, 29, 65, 219, 238
    financial analysis in, 59–60, 202, 229–30
    management of, 15, 19, 56–57
    mergers in, 56, 59
    number of, 57
    profit in, 91, 202–3, 229–31
    race to market in, 16, 35–36, 84
    R&D investment, 89–91
    sales reps, 81–82, 190, 205
    scenario without Amendments, 209–11, 232–39
    small firms. *See* small drug companies
    university collaboration with, 79, 105–6

Pharmaceutical Manufacturers' Association (PMA), 14, 58–59
Pharmaceutical Research and Manufacturing Association (PhRMA), 58–59
pharmacies
    compounding, 93–95
    drug prices in. *See* prices
Phase 1 trials, 51
Phase 2 trials, 51
Phase 3 trials, 51–54, 193
Phase 4 trials, 55, 87
phocomelia, 9
PhRMA. *See* Pharmaceutical Research and Manufacturing Association (PhRMA)
physicians. *See also specific physicians*
    FDA bias against, 132–33, 176–77
    information sources, 226
    innovation by
        cancer treatments, 132–37, 203, 236
        stem cell research, 127–31, 203
    knowledge about natural products, 124, 169, 190, 204–5
    nutrition information for, 169–70
    off-label information for, 81–82, 205
placebo effect
    defined, 24
    effectiveness and, 140
    ethical issues with, 63, 69, 77, 233
plasma, freeze-dried, 219–20
PMA. *See* Pharmaceutical Manufacturers' Association (PMA)
Pneumocystis pneumonia (PCP), 69–71

pneumonia, 69–71, 101–2

political influences, 61–72, 148–54

polychlorinated biphenyls (PCBs), 190

post-approval studies, 38, 55, 87

preclinical work, 48–51, 96. *See also* animal testing

pregnancy
folic acid, 3, 163–65, 180, 204, 230
labor induction, 196
premature births, 93–95
thalidomide tragedy, 1, 3, 9–10, 25, 145, 212

premarket notification, 194

premature births, 93–95

Prescription Drug User Fee Act (PD-UFA), 30, 140–41, 150–52, 180, 202–4, 236

President's Biomedical Research Panel, 40

prevention
information about, 171–74
scenario without Amendments, 209–11, 237–38
versus treatment. *See* paradigm shift

prices
cartelization and, 58–59
effect of development costs on, 50, 54, 88–96, 235–36, 301
generic drugs, 97–100
of natural products, 211
of drugs without the Amendments, 91–96, 210–11, 235–36

pro-drugs, 189–91

product reviews, 223–28, 230

profit, 91, 202–3, 229–31

progesterone, 93–95

propranolol, 39–40, 81

prostacyclin (PGI$_2$), 76–77

prostaglandins
aspirin's effect on, 76–79
from burn cream, 172–74
cytoprotective, 149
for gastric ulcers, 154–55
for liver disease, 107–9, 111, 113, 122
patent for, 159

prostaglandin E$_1$ (PGE1), 195–96

prostate cancer, 117–20

Provenge, 117–20

Proxmire, William, 179–80

PRRT. *See* Peptide Receptor Radionuclide Therapy (PRRT)

PSA, 117

psychotropic drugs, 41

publications, 225

Public Citizens, 227

Pyridorin˙, 193

pyridoxamine dihydrochloride, 192–93

Q

quality of life, 46, 126

R

Raab, G. Kirk, 18

radiation damage, 172–74

rattlesnake oil, 231

RDAs. *See* recommended daily allowances (RDAs)

recombinant human insulin, 30–31

recombinant proteins, 41

recommended daily allowances (RDAs), 159, 167

regulations. *See also specific law*
   versus certification, 222–28
   costs of, 205–6, 212–13
regulatory review time
   generic drugs, 97
   new indications, 82, 147
   patents and, 74
   political influences on, 61–72, 148–54
research. *See also* testing
   versus development, 79, 105–6, 203
   efficiency of, 96
respiratory syncytial virus (RSV), 66
ribavirin, 32, 66–68
Richardson-Merrell, 9, 144
rickets, 166–67
"Right to Try" legislation, 219
risk-to-benefit assessment, 27
Robert, André, 154–55
robotics, 96
Rogaine®, 171–72
Rorvik, David, 132
Rothschild, Nathan, 101
RSV. *See* respiratory syncytial virus (RSV)

afety
   animal studies. *See* animal testing
   approvals as guarantee of, 26, 28–31, 198, 213–14
   effect of Amendments on, 140–41, 146–48, 201
   "safe for their intended use," 9
   side effects, 143–44, 146–56
salicin, 231

Salk polio vaccine, 143–45
Sanofi, 99
Sarepta, 232–35
Schmidt, Alexander, 115
Schwartzman, David, 113
Seal of Approval, 223, 226
Sears, Barry, 79
sea snake oil, 231
Shaw, Sandy, 218
Shilts, Randy, 68
shingles, 82
Shkreli, Martin, 98
side effects, 143–44, 146–56. *See also* safety; *specific drugs*
skin cream, 172–74
small drug companies. *See also specific companies*
   cartelization and, 57–69, 197–98, 202–3, 210, 213
   innovation by, 117–20
   price gouging by, 56–60, 203
   scenario without Amendments, 210, 232–35
snake oil, 231
Sobel, Russell S., 24
Sofer, Gideon J., 37
Somers, Suzanne, 130, 177
Spain, 142
Spencer, Leslie, 18
spina bifida, 3, 163–65, 180, 204, 230
split-label approach, 218
Squibb Chemical Company, 75, 77, 80
Staphage lifsate, 132
statins, 186–87
statistical analysis and significance, 52–54, 96, 108, 118

stem cell research, 127–31, 203, 238
Stewart, William, 102
stock options, 59–60, 202, 229–30
stomach ulcers, 124, 149, 154–55
stroke, 44, 75, 79, 148
sunlight, 167
superbugs, 13, 102–3
Supreme Court, 15, 23–24, 28, 36. *See also* court rulings
surrogate markers, 65–66, 96, 108
Syntex, 69

T
Tahoma Clinic (WA), 176–77
Takeda, 20–21
television advertising, 26, 91, 221
terminally ill patients, 19–21, 35–37, 200, 219
testing
    animal. *See* animal testing
    automation of, 96
    bioequivalence studies, 97
    efficiency of, 95–96
    human. *See* human studies
    scenario without Amendments, 236–37
    third-party, 223–28
    US-based requirement, 41, 52, 62
    in vitro, 48–49, 96
testosterone, 93–95
Teva, 99
Texas, 134–36, 175–76
thalidomide
    birth defects caused by, 1, 3, 9–10, 25, 144–45, 212
    FDA approval of, 195–96
third-party testing, 223–28

thromboxane (TxB$_2$), 76–77
Todd, James, 63
toxicology testing. *See* animal testing
toxoplasmosis, 98–99
trade secrets, 57
transplantation, 195
"treatment INDs," 35–37
treatment versus prevention. *See* paradigm shift
triglycerides, 190
tuberculosis, 101–2
Tufts University, 112–14
Turing Pharmaceuticals, 98
TxB$_2$. *See* thromboxane (TxB$_2$)
Tylenol, 188

U
UL Seal of Approval, 223
ultraviolet light, 167
Underwriters Laboratories (UL), 223
United Kingdom
    drug development in
        cost of, 39
        time required for, 38–39, 142
    drug prices in, 58
    Duchenne's disease drugs in, 233, 235
    innovation in, 115–16, 142
    number of new drugs in, 39–41 142
    regulatory approach in, 38, 55 141–42
university research, 79, 105–6. *See also specific universities*
Upjohn Company
    anti-anxiety drugs, 51
    anti-oxidants, 161–62

aspirin, 76–79

attitude toward regulatory demands, 47

development decisions at, 73, 160

focus on costs, 103–4

gastric ulcer research, 154–55

LD50 testing at, 49

liver disease research, 107–9, 111, 113, 122

minoxidil, 171–72

Motrin, 149

motto of, 144

nutrition research, 157–58

Panalba, 13–15, 103–4

PGE1, 195–96

size of, 57

Upjohn, W. E., 144

US Congress. *See* Congress

US Constitution, First Amendment, 29, 55, 82, 171, 180

US Defense Department, 219–20

user fees, 30, 140–41, 150–52, 180, 202–4, 236

US Office of Technology Assessment, 86

V

vaccines, 41, 143–45

Valeant Pharmaceuticals International, 120

Vascepa, 190

Viagra, 196

Vioxx, 148–56, 209, 229–30

viral hepatitis, 108–9

vitamins, 158–59, 166

vitamin B6, 192–93

vitamin D, 166–70, 204

vitamin E, 161–62

W

Wall Street Journal, 117

walnuts, 184–85

Wardell, William M., 123

warning letters (FDA), 182–85

Washington, 176–77

Waxman Hatch Patent Restoration Act, 74, 236

Weidenbaum, Murray, 210

Weinberg, John, 176

whistleblowers, 5–6, 17, 21

willow bark, 231

withdrawal

from development, 55, 86, 91, 108–9, 113–14, 121–22, 140–42

from market, 15, 152, 214

Woodroof, Ron, 33

Worst Pills, Best Pills (newsletter), 227

Wright, Jonathan, 176–77

Y

Young, Frank, 32, 67, 208

Z

Zone Diet, 79

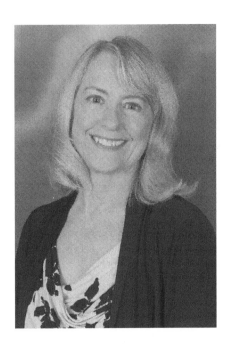

Dr. Mary J. Ruwart is a research scientist, ethicist, and author. She received her BS in biochemistry in 1970 and her PhD in biophysics in 1974 (both from Michigan State University). She subsequently joined the Department of Surgery at St. Louis University as a post-doctoral student and was subsequently promoted to instructor and assistant professor of surgery there. She left in 1976 to accept a position with The Upjohn Company of Kalamazoo, Michigan. As a senior research scientist, Ruwart was involved in developing new therapies for a variety of diseases, including liver cirrhosis and AIDS.

Ruwart left Upjohn in 1995 to devote her time to teaching, consulting, and writing. Between 2003 and 2006, she was an adjunct associate professor of biology at the University of North Carolina in Charlotte. During that time, she served with the Center for Applied and Professional Ethics, designing a medical research ethics course for the university. Her radical application of ethics to medical regulation, especially regulations regarding pharmaceuticals, has life-and-death implications. Ruwart provides consulting services for nutraceutical companies, clinical research organizations, and universities and expert testimony in FDA-related cases. She currently chairs a for-profit IRB (Institutional Review Board) in the Austin area.

Dr. Ruwart also is chair of Liberty International (https://liberty-intl
org/), secretary of the Foundation for a Free Society (https://www
acebook.com/myfreesociety), and health care advisor to the Heartland
nstitute (https://www.heartland.org/index.html). She can be reached
hrough her website at http://www.ruwart.com.

*   *   *

You can communicate with the author at http://www.ruwart.com. By
sing coupon code "deathbyregulation," you can get a $5 savings on any
tem on her website.